MENTORING, PRECEPTORSHIP AND CLINICAL SUPERVISION

A Guide to Professional Support Roles in Clinical Practice

Second Edition

ALISON MORTON-COOPER
PhD, MEd, RN

and

ANNE PALMER
MA, BEd (Hons), RN, RM, RNT

Blackwell
Science

Blackwell Science Ltd, a Blackwell Publishing company
Editorial offices:
Blackwell Science Ltd, 9600 Garsington Road, Oxford OX4 2DQ, UK
    Tel: +44 (0) 1865 776868
Blackwell Publishing Inc., 350 Main Street, Malden, MA 02148-5020, USA
    Tel: +1 781 388 8250
Blackwell Science Asia Pty Ltd, 550 Swanston Street, Carlton, Victoria 3053, Australia
    Tel: +61 (0)3 8359 1011

First published 1993
Reprinted 1994, 1995, 1996
Second edition published 2000
Reprinted 2001, 2002, 2003, 2005

Library of Congress Cataloging-in-Publication Data
Morton-Cooper, Alison.
    Mentoring, preceptorship, and clinical supervision :
    a guide to professional roles in clinical practice /
    Alison Morton-Cooper and Anne
    Palmer.–2nd ed.
        p.   cm.
    Rev. ed. of: Mentoring and
    preceptorship. c1998
    Includes bibliographical references
    and indexes.
        ISBN 0-632-04967-7 (pb)
        1. Mentoring in nursing–Great Britain.
    Nursing–Study and teaching
    (Preceptorship)–Great Britain.
    I. Palmer, Anne. II. Morton–Cooper,
    Alison. Mentoring and preceptorship.
    III. Title.
        [DNLM: 1. Education, Nursing–
    methods. 2. Clinical Competence.
    3. Mentors. 4. Nursing, Supervisory.
    5. Preceptorship. WY 18.5 M889ma 2000]
    RT86.45 .M67 2000
    610.78'071'55–dc21 99-086121

ISBN-10: 0-632-04967-7
ISBN-13: 978-0632-04967-7

A catalogue record for this title is available from the British Library

Set in 10/12.5pt Century Book
by DP Photosetting, Aylesbury, Bucks
Printed and bound by Replika Press Pvt. Ltd, India

For further information on Blackwell Publishing, visit our website:
www.blackwellpublishing.com

For all those who are learning,
reflecting and supporting in practice.

About the Authors

Alison Morton-Cooper is an experienced researcher-practitioner specialising in organisational learning and development. She is currently Lecturer in Health Studies at the University of Glasgow (Crichton campus, Dumfries) and Associate Fellow in Continuing Education at the University of Warwick.

Ann Palmer is director of post-graduate studies, Centre for Community Care and Primary Health, University of Westminster, and a part-time education consultant with extensive experience of teaching and learning in health care.

Contents

Foreword

Malcolm Tight
Professor of Continuing Education
University of Warwick

I always feel a mixture of emotions when I am asked to do something like this: write a foreword for a book, chair a conference session, provide a job reference, review a paper for a journal. Pleasure and challenge are the most prominent amongst them. Pleasure because it is always nice to be asked, it isn't a particularly onerous task and it is pleasing to be associated in this way with both the authors and the book. Challenge, because I then wonder what I might or should say. There is an unspoken and unwritten etiquette about these things.

My own special interest is in higher education policy and practice and I also teach in the broader territories of adult/continuing/lifelong education and learning, subjects which lie at the centre of the professional education and learning debate.

One-to-one relationships of the kind described in this book are undeniably of critical importance in the professional development of the individual. They are also, by their very nature, varied and individualised. In twenty years in academia I have personally survived largely unmentored, or at least not as these authors would define 'true mentoring' (see p 46). I only experienced a *pseudo*-mentoring relationship, rarely and without the sustained nurturing true mentoring can encourage. Perhaps if I had received better support at critical points in my academic career I could have travelled differently or with a different perspective.

It is only in the last few years that mentoring has begun to be formalised in institutions such as mine and it is still the case, in many walks of life, that receiving comprehensive professional learning support remains unusual. It is therefore very refreshing for me to learn about the development of such systems and to see how it can enhance the experience of lifelong learning and of 'becoming professional'.

The simple fact that this is the second edition of this book illustrates how well Alison's and Anne's work has been received. Clearly, there are many people out there who have already benefited from the ideas contained here. This second edition remains a potent mixture of theory, practice and advice, suitably updated and expanded.

Whether you dive in to the sections that particularly interest you, or immerse yourself in the book as a whole, will depend upon your needs and circumstances. But do engage with the experience and suggestions presented, and enjoy the stimulation they provide. This is a rare book: theoretical, practical and well-written.

Preface

Introducing professional learning support systems into clinical practice is a major issue for today's health professionals. This book aims to help practitioners faced with the challenge of turning study and work into a dynamic and engaging learning environment by guiding them through the maze of concepts and ideas which have emerged in learning support in recent years. It also shows how the appropriate use of concepts can greatly enhance the quality of life for practitioners and patients.

All health professionals are warmly welcomed to participate in the debate which we entered into as authors in the first edition of the book, and which many readers and practitioners have refined, developed and moved forward in the intervening years.

As practitioners take on the demands of lifelong learning in the workplace, educators and employers have a responsibility to see that workable support systems provide the right stimulus for role learning and the acquisition of professional skills. Learning can then be viewed as a pleasurable challenge and an opportunity to build on professional values as part of a developing portfolio of professional expertise.

We believe that, to be taken seriously, learning support practice must first be underpinned by sound conceptual and theoretical analysis. Without this, support concepts are merely reduced to the latest 'buzz-words' and passing fads in an era which looks to soundbites for policy formation in public service provision. Health professionals need and deserve support systems which recognise and value their important contribution to the health of the nation, and which help to build trust and collegiality in the workplace.

This book therefore aims high, hoping to make sound pragmatic sense to practitioners while making sure that the models of learning support they propose are theoretically sound. We anticipate that readers will want to use the book in a variety of ways:

- As a textbook for courses on teaching, learning and assessment
- As part of formal preparation for undertaking support roles in practice
- When an in-depth analysis of support issues is needed for strategic planning purposes
- For practice development and project work

- As a contribution to the literature on mentoring, preceptorship and clinical supervision.

The first chapter examines the contemporary context of health care work from a sociological perspective and looks at the impact our work roles have on our relationships and life experiences. It discusses the personal and professional demands made on practitioners and argues that formal learning support systems are becoming essential to our collective well-being.

Chapter 2 introduces and explores the concept of mentoring from its probable origins in ancient Greece and considers its applications and different meanings in a variety of settings, including business, general education and applied health care. The focus is that of the 'classical mentor' and how this role has been interpreted through history and by differing organisational challenges and demands. Enabling characteristics are then identified, explored and modified so as to separate the distinguishing characteristics of mentoring from those of other professional support roles in practice. The chapter goes on to examine the ways in which mentoring systems and processes may be developed for practice both formally and informally. Case studies are also offered to bring alive the 'lived experience' of mentoring.

Chapter 3 explains why the introduction of preceptorship has had a variable impact on learning support in clinical practice and why it is as yet under-developed as a means of helping practitioners to manage career transitions effectively. The outcomes of a practice-based doctoral study on the implementation of preceptorship in British nursing are published for the first time in this chapter, together with criteria for effective preceptorship which were developed by practitioners as important corollaries of the study. The findings graphically illustrate some of the problems practitioners experience when trying to introduce elements of transitional learning support into practice and they raise issues of interest and concern to practitioners and policymakers alike.

Clinical supervision is currently high on the nursing agenda in Britain and much has been written about this emerging professional support role in recent years. Authors and researchers have grappled with developing models, extolled the benefits and begun to identify its limitations. Chapter 4 continues the debate by decoding the language of clinical supervision and addressing relevant issues for practice.

Chapter 5 draws the book to a close by offering a glossary of support roles and by presenting an overall framework for professional learning support. The practicalities of implementing and undertaking professional roles are considered, along with some of the ethical issues involved. Most importantly, this chapter aims to compare the roles of mentor, preceptor and clinical supervisor and to tease out the differences between them based on our own studies and considerable professional experience.

This second edition is opportune and timely in being published just as the health care professions are made aware of the important and far-reaching recommendations announced by the UKCC's Commission on Nursing & Midwifery Education (1999). Entitled *Fitness for Practice,** the commission makes no bones about the centrality of professional learning support to ensuring fitness for practice and at least six of the Commission's recommendations address mentoring, preceptorship and clinical supervision directly.

In order to raise and improve standards of professional practice, higher education institutions and service providers alike are exhorted to make sure that:

- students, assessors and mentors know what is expected of them through specified outcomes and competencies which form part of a formal learning contract (recommendation 13);
- a period of supervised clinical practice of at least three months duration is provided towards the end of the pre-registration programme (20);
- all newly qualified registrants should receive a properly supported period of induction and preceptorship when they begin their employment (21);
- the preparation, support and feedback to mentors and preceptors is properly formalised (28);
- funding to support learning in practice should take account of the cost of mentoring, assessment by clinical staff, and lecturers having regular contact with practice (29);
- the health care professions should actively be encouraged to learn from one another (32).

We are none of us left in any doubt, then, that formal professional learning support systems have a crucial role to play in the development and maintenance of safe and effective health care practice.

For us, this book is part of the necessary evolution of professional learning support and as such is clearly open to critical analysis and contention. The move towards interprofessional and collaborative working will provide many opportunities for health professionals to engage meaningfully in the continuing debate and we look forward to sharing in this as we look to the future.

Alison Morton-Cooper and Anne Palmer
October 1999

*UKCC (1999) *Fitness for Practice – the UKCC Commission for Nursing and Midwifery Education,* London, United Kingdom Central Council for Nursing, Midwifery & Health Visiting.

Acknowledgements

I would like to take this opportunity to thank the Kathleen Blundell Trust (administered by the Society of Authors) whose generous financial assistance has allowed me to undertake valuable comparative studies on preceptorship in the USA. The strategic and financial support of the former West Midlands Regional Health Authority, England, in helping me to examine policy and practice in professional learning support is also gratefully acknowledged.

Sincere thanks is extended to all of the practitioners and academics whose involvement, enthusiasm, honesty and integrity has greatly enriched my studies since the first edition of this book was published. Thanks are also due to the staff of the Royal College of Nursing Library, Edinburgh, for practical advice and assistance.

Alison Morton-Cooper

It is always a pleasure to sit back when the hard graft is nearly over and consider those who have sustained the reflective endeavours and made them enjoyable. I am grateful to all those who stimulated my thought processes and influenced my practice over the years and I remain indebted to the individuals I identified in the first edition.

This time around I am particularly grateful to Jude Hanner – for providing a safe haven, Debra Humphris – for the conceptual pragmatism and friendship, Roger Pietroni and Ros Freeman for offering a different dimension and to Brigid Proctor for stimulating my grey cells. I also extend thanks to all those I am still working and learning with – my colleagues and students at the University of Westminster, my friends at the SOLAR Centre, Nene University College and everyone at Educare Consulting. I also wish to acknowledge my mother who started my learning journey and who is learning to live with Alzheimer's disease with dignity and humour. I could not manage without the team at the Kingshill Research Centre or the staff at Langton House in Wiltshire – you all do a brilliant job under difficult conditions. Finally, this second edition would not have been achieved without the gentle cajoling of a first class publisher, Griselda Campbell, and the supportive administration of Rebecca Stevens.

Anne Palmer

Chapter 1
The Context of Health Care Work

Trust and dependence in health care organisations

Who are we and what are we doing here? In the *busy*ness of being health professionals we seldom afford the time to ask ourselves the bigger questions. Perhaps this is because we perceive these questions as too big to contemplate. Working in a culture which seems to prize toughness and resilience over other personal qualities, we think it is better to get on and do, rather than to stop and reflect on what is happening to us and why, or what impact our contribution is making to the lives of people whom we care for, communicate with, exert control over or make value judgements about.

When we try to make sense of the puzzles and uncertainties of daily life we do so from a highly interpretive perspective:

> 'We tend to interpret the uncertainties of everyday life in terms of our self-doubts, rather than the social structures which condition them. We imagine that if we were cleverer, more educated, less shy, or more attractive, we would be as secure and confident as other people appear to be; and because each of us is hiding this sense of personal inadequacy, we are slow to discover how pervasively our culture induces these feelings.'

(Marris, 1996, p. 12)

Such are the insecurities of our social relationships that we seek out explanations for our inadequacy in 'the system' some of the time and in ourselves at others. In trying to atone for our perceived failings we succumb to what has been described as the 'performance culture' (Davies, 1995), a culture of work which seeks to test out whether we are good enough, professionally and personally, to do the jobs we are paid to do.

What we do not – perhaps cannot – always appreciate is the wider social picture, the fact that we may be but a microcosm of a much broader social structure, a structure and a collective which is struggling to adapt on a grander scale to ever-burgeoning demands on limited resources.

Many of the policy debates and initiatives which focus on performance, on standards, benchmarks and league tables, can appear to leech away at the 'added value' of our commitment to caring professionally, and for some, threaten the ethos of trust within the workplace. This leads us to another difficult question. If we cannot trust and rely on each other, then to whom can we turn when the challenges overwhelm us? Such anxieties run deep and we develop strategies for dealing with them:

> 'This tendency to blame oneself for the world's ills is itself a strategy for mastering uncertainty. To change one's own behaviour, to learn to fit in better, is less daunting and more immediately practical than to reform the structure of social relationships: and to mistrust oneself is less frightening than to see clearly how dangerously untrustworthy the societies we inhabit may be.'

> (Marris, 1996, p. 12)

The idea that we are alone and unsupported would for many of us be too hard to accept. Swirling in the maelstrom of political, organisational and cultural change, it seems that health professionals have seldom been confronted by so many competing demands. The quest to restore order and to find meaning and significance in what we do which transcends the language and culture of performance is frequently expressed both openly and covertly. But there also appears to be a feeling that the personal consequences of the work we do for our emotional and family lives is seldom considered, at least not in any overt way.

The risks we take and the ways in which we are made vulnerable are many and varied. Some are more visible and tangible than others. Marris believes that our capacity to adapt and survive such challenges to our personal stability exists in our thoughts and actions. The values which we hand down from one generation to the next become embodied in our institutions (family, church, workplace, profession, leisure activities) to become 'systems of relationship which express ... meanings and reproduce them' and it is the manipulation of such meaning which exerts power over us (Marris, 1996, p. 20–23).

In striving for perfection, professionals try hard to contain their own anxieties and vulnerabilities. Care professionals may themselves start from a base of wanting to feel loved, to belong and to be appreciated, but there is little opportunity to address the frustrations of the work we do. Barber describes the problem graphically:

'Outlets for distress are usually blocked by the working culture. The person within the professional role learns to cope by splitting emotions off from the intellect, thus repressing painful experiences.'

(Barber, 1996, p. 63)

Displacement of personal distress is thus characterised as 'workaholism', in strategies such as 'fighting bad feelings upon the inside with good works on the outside' or in obsessionally working to rules, all of which, Barber points out (1996, p. 63), is ultimately unsuccessful in taking the core hurt away. In trying to 'grapple with uncertainty, to make the world predictable enough to act purposefully in it, we adapt to our own experience the ways of seeing and of thinking about what we see . . .' (Marris, 1996 p. 25). Our personal beliefs, prejudices, ideals, and worries inform our behaviour and our judgements regarding the behaviours of others, others' defences against uncertainty being much more obvious to us than our own.

This second edition of a book which attempts to explore and outline strategies of social support which can help us to learn with and from each other is therefore very much a product of its time. Our defences against the disillusionment, dissatisfaction and sense of inadequacy in meeting the perceived standards others expect of us require close and critical examination of the ways in which we perceive and characterise our personal and collective 'enemies'. Lack of time, too many managers and too little money are all strong candidates.

In the previous edition we outlined our personal interpretation and vision of how we felt support roles could mediate against the potentially damaging effects of working in a physically and psychologically demanding culture. In the six years which have elapsed since then, it has been made clear to us how all-embracing the feeling of personal vulnerability is both in terms of the individual and in the collegial cultures which have grown up around the various health disciplines. The shared experience of responding to needs and framing health services, has, in some ways, brought professionals closer together while in others it has driven a wedge – an apparent competitiveness and protectionist reponse to perceived encroachments on our professional 'territories'.

For this reason, as authors with a background in nursing, higher education and human resource development, we have chosen to take a generic interprofessional approach to the subject of learning support in health care. We hope this will reflect the very valuable contributions made to the book by the many students and seasoned professionals of all disciplines who have added to and enriched our understanding of the apparent motivational crisis which is currently affecting health care professionals in the UK.

In the chapters which follow we look closely at the ways in which learning support can be used to help restore meaning and a sense of emotional security between and for colleagues, all of whom are ostensibly working towards the same goal of better health services for all.

The emerging crisis of trust in public services

Part of the difficulty inherent in professional health care work is the drive towards professional autonomy in the face of (at least for NHS workers) hierarchical top–down organisation (Rogers *et al.*, 1999, p. 86). The problem for nurses is particularly well documented:

> 'Emotionally and psychologically, nursing is a difficult job at the best of times; nurses confront serious illness, death and disability every day, as well as the fear and pain felt by every patient. They have to deal with distressed relatives and friends, and to cope with their own sense of loss and pain. Over time they become accustomed to the feelings, sights, sounds and smells, but they do not necessarily learn to handle them constructively, either for themselves or for others. If they do learn to do so, it is often through their own efforts rather than those of the system, which offers too little preparation, education and support.'

> (Rogers *et al.*, 1999, p. 84)

It is difficult to grasp the scale of the support problem for all staff in health care. There is good reason to speculate that we have documented only the tip of the iceberg when it comes to the support needs of staff working in health care services (see Borrill *et al.* 1996, 1998).

Even patients and clients are remarkably under-supported when it comes to dealing with the emotional and psychological fall-out of being on the receiving end of professional care. Medical anthropologists who set out to provide authentic accounts of what it feels like to be ill have difficulty in finding studies which adequately portray the experience of being unwell and at the mercy of health care providers (Good, 1994, p. 117). Accounts of what it is like to *care for* people are therefore at least some kind of useful progress on what it means to be vulnerable and human in the health care scenario.

In a recently reported large scale study on stress among staff in 19 NHS Trusts in England, researchers at Sheffield University's Institute of Work Psychology found that managers were most affected by stress, with ancillary workers describing the fewest effects. When compared with workers in other equivalent professional groups in the general population, the stress levels of nurses were described as 40% higher. NHS staff as a whole fared poorly when compared with British employees generally (Borrill *et al.*, 1996, 1998).

The mass media's tendency to frame discussions and reportage of health care problems in 'crisis' terms, together with highly publicised and emotive developments in central government's attempts to make health professionals more accountable, cannot help to contain the feelings of dissatisfaction and discontent with health care work which have already come to prominence in the professional literature. Public confidence in the reliability and efficacy of services is also challenged daily with the increase in litigation for faults in the system and the problems generated by greater reliance on sophisticated medical technology rather than traditional care-giving. The distinction between care and cure is, as ever, a blurred one for patients and is perhaps the reason why demands for effective advocacy of patients are increasing (e.g. Teasdale, 1998).

Staff at the so-called sharp end of care-giving, therefore, have a number of problems to deal with on a daily basis. The multiple and diverse demands of patients, relatives, managers, professional colleagues and the 'public interest' have somehow to be reconciled with the professional's self-image and self-expectation of what it is to be an ethical and conscientious care provider within the context of health work.

Learning to live with uncertainty

Marris argues that in learning to live with uncertainty we have to establish some shared understandings of what it means to co-exist with others. In his view, the meanings we attach to significant events and people in our lives are therefore what hold us together in the individual management of uncertainty. In the nurturing of our relationships and our ability to develop shared, meaningful understandings lies our best hope for the future.

Our forms of *attachment* to each other can help to build trust and a mutual sense of purposeful direction. The lack of such attachment to each other is for some sociologists very characteristic of work in the 'new capitalism' of the third millennium, with 'here today, gone tomorrow' philosophies coming to represent the experience of people attempting to come to terms with the global culture of economic determinism which pervaded the culture of work at the end of the twentieth century, at least in western societies (Sennett, 1998).

High turnover of staff and patients within a cost-led rather than demand-led service can leave employees who work in a service culture with an undeniable sense of conflict of interest. Health professionals who are expected to fulfil the demands of both employer and patient are thus prone to feelings of guilt and inadequacy. The need to 'fit in' with the prevailing culture in order to survive can lead to strong feelings of internal conflict and a sense of moral anxiety over the right course of action to take in day-to-day situations (Holden, 1991).

The consequences of poor staff morale, a sense of being under-valued by society, the proliferation of other less personally demanding/more rewarding career opportunities and less flexible working practices for health workers, must have contributed significantly to the rise in recruitment and rentention problems experienced by health care employers in recent years.

The emotional needs of carers are clear. For nurses it is said to be the acknowledged and unacknowledged need to be a person, to be seen to be doing something good and to be able to say, at the end of the day, that the world is a better place because of their contribution:

> 'The needs to be acknowledged as a person are deep and real, and are often confusing and get in the way of caring. When they are understood and given a name they are no longer threatening, but become tools for working with and achieving great things. However, if they are unacknowledged they can deteriorate and wreak havoc.'

> (Tschudin, 1997, p. 158)

The many personal and psychological risks inherent in health care work – from industrial injury to psychological distress – represent a huge challenge to health service employers, the NHS having no better record for managing employees' health needs than any other employer (Rogers *et al.*, 1999). The personal and collective consequences of health care work can therefore result in a lack of psychological and social commitment and attachment in the institutional contexts of health care work. Trust between employer and employee is prone to breakdown, with a rise in feelings of helplessness, cynicism and unwillingness to make further psychological or emotional investments in the outcomes of health related employment.

The other chapters in this book address some of these deep-seated and heart-felt insecurities by tackling head-on the root causes of our anxiety and conflict in learning about and providing high standards of care. The ability to not just survive, but *thrive* in such a culture is the over-arching theme of this book.

Identifying and developing a culture of secure attachment and trust within health care work may seem highly idealistic and ambitious, we know, but we recognise from our own involvement in the system that such ideals are attainable, *provided* we work together and develop shared and mutually meaningful understandings of what it is we are trying to achieve.

Trust and 'relations of support'

Trust between people is a social virtue. It permeates all relationships and is vital to organisations because, like families, organisations amount to social entities or they are nothing (Herriot *et al.*, 1998, p. 47). Without the society constituted by people there would be no point in the existence of a health care system.

The cultural consequences of inadequate support systems are evident in the accounts provided by health workers of the psychological and physical strains placed on them. The vulnerability of the medical student is made clear in the account described in Box 1.1.

Box 1.1.

'For the young medical student who is well into the energy-consuming processes of the personal development necessary for his [sic] age, and whose life is devoid of adequate supports or the strength derived from experience, there flows a succession of other people's distressing feelings and the raw emotions of his chosen career.

These seem to pack themselves into his day, one on top of another, too fast to contemplate, and so many, so fast, demand he distance himself behind the white coat of one who may be presumed to prevent death. He is pressured to join a club of people whose membership enables him to enter the hospital wards not as a patient – a person who can be ill, disabled or in pain – but quite, quite separate, as 'doctor'. He puts on a cloak of defence against human emotions, which too frequently also separates him from his own tender growth and sensitivity.'

(Holland, 1995, p. 14)

The idea that trust is reciprocal, and that relationships of trust require each party involved to fulfil obligations to one another, is characteristic of the *psychological contract* between employer and employee, patient and carer, colleagues and friends. For health care professionals there is the additional (perceived?) burden of the *service ideal*, which is based on the belief that 'professional action should be based on the needs of the client alone, and not the needs of the professional nor even those of society' (Eraut, 1994 p. 225). As Eraut advises, historically the assumption has been that because of their specialist knowledge it is only the professionals who can decide what the clients' needs are, a position which is increasingly being challenged in the public domain as concepts such as clients' rights and choice are examined and articulated.

The demand for greater public accountability requires that professionals no longer have the monopoly on deciding what patients' or clients' needs are, but that they become only one possible provider of these needs. Other issues to do with equity, rationing and political acceptability also enter the picture.

Legal (if imperfect) frameworks exist to protect the vulnerable public from the incompetence of professionals. Few effective frameworks (legal or otherwise), however, exist to protect employees from the destabilising emotional impact caused by trying to reconcile the ideals of professional practice with the harsh economic realities of what professionals can provide.

The sociologist Abigayl Perry provides an excellent example of the effects of competing demands on the health and well-being of employees (see Box 1.2.).

Box 1.2

'Doctors need clever pairs of hands to assist them in their technical tasks. Hospital administrators need well-regimented pairs of feet which respond in uniform ways to different marching orders and constant changes in battle plans. Patients need human compassion, carers who respect them as persons and not merely as bodies.

All these groups want what money in a money economy does not necessarily buy. They want the *love* of worker bees, with their dedication of purpose, superb instincts and organisational skills. Who tries to live up to these impossibly high and unstated expectations in human caring and who therefore suffers the personal consequences of failing to meet these needs? Usually nurses in health care and usually women in the family and society generally.'

(Perry, 1993, p. 62)

It would not be unfair, given accounts such as these, to view health care systems as forming a 'low trust society', a system which fails to sustain itself adequately in the face of such overwhelming demands (see Fukuyama (1996) for a discussion on the economic and social impact of a 'low trust' society.)

Trust and the value of education

Our ability to survive relies on what remains of trust and mutual dependency within the organisations and settings in which we work, be they institutional or community based. The value of education in helping people to 'systematically unveil the lines of dependency' affecting their existence is well recognised if not always acted out in our workplaces and communities (Hart, 1992, p. 200) As a fairly radical exponent of what education in adulthood can do to promote better relations of support, Hart challenges us to respond to the needs of individuals to make better sense of their predicaments by asking critical and much needed questions. She believes that adult educators (and we would interpret this as anyone with an interest in learning in the workplace) need to let go of the fixation we have on 'merely building a quality workforce which will contribute to effectiveness:'

'Adult education would have to see the current troubled experiences of work, accompanied by doubts, problems, dissatisfactions and sufferings as an opportunity for asking critical questions, and for opening up at least the conception of new possibilities for living and working. To feel the pulse of these kinds of changes, to be a midwife to these unborn ideas, to articulate them and give them means of social expression which would make them conscious and actionable – this should be an educational task of primary importance.'

(Hart, 1992, p. 200)

Hart argues that current and developing forms of workplace organisation tend to destroy the last vestiges of what she describes as a 'work-related social culture', despite their emphasis on teams and other collaborative forms of work. For her, the fault lies in their top–down origins, with such forms of work being 'instituted from above'. Instead, Hart would like to see workers exploring new ways of creating work environments where individual workers can rely on mutual support and encouragement, 'thereby strengthening the attempts to shape this environment in accordance with worker-defined needs and interests.' (Hart, 1992, p. 206).

The concept of *critical thinking* is therefore a central one, with the aim of increasing worker democracy and *relations of support* in work organisations as espoused by Brookfield (1987). Critical thinkers actively involve themselves in developing a vision of how things could be, rather than how they are.

'Critical thinkers see the future as open and malleable, not as closed and fixed. They are self-confident about their potential for changing aspects of their worlds, both as individuals and through collective action'.

(Brookfield, 1987, 4-5)

Possibilities for re-evaluating and challenging our lot as health professionals therefore include asking critical questions about the *status quo*, not simply in order to explain our experiences, but also to formulate some kind of action for changing what we want to change, and for re-negotiating our positions from our particular standpoints.

Different health disciplines are thought to enjoy different levels of power and respect in organisations, and the ways in which these power relations are interpreted can have a significant impact on the confidence and readiness of different health care workers to challenge their perceived influence within hierarchical organisations. We would argue that the concept of *stress*, for example, and the language which has come to dominate the ways in which we think about and deal with stress, are largely responsible for a feeling of learned helplessness among some health professionals.

Our lack of control over the work situation and our feelings of insecurity about the worth of our contribution to health care as professional care-givers is culturally mediated, with some professionals feeling more powerful (and therefore more valued) than others, at both the level of individuals and from a professional perspective. The wholesale adoption of the stress discourse into the culture of the workplace has profound implications for our ability to devise effective support frameworks for ourselves, and for our abilities to make employers recognise the need to support us meaningfully in our enterprise.

Discourse, or the language we use to explain and explore our understandings, is a powerful medium. Without it, human beings would have to design completely new ways of communicating needs and concerns to one another. *Discourse analysis* is a means by which social scientists seek to understand the way people build or 'construct their own realities' about situations as they see them. In examining the discourse of *work-related stress*, for example, we refer here to the psycho-social effects on the workplace culture of accepting and reproducing ideas about stress without critically examining what the concept really means for us as individuals and employees.

Does our everyday social use of the concept of stress actually help us to bear our load more evenly? Does it make us feel more confident about our chances of dealing with the demands made on us? Previous generations worried about whether their crops might fail, feared the effects of flood and plague, had fewer concerns about the individualistic nature of being alive, their main objective being to survive against different and often unpredictable odds.

It is not uncommon to hear senior citizens decry the concept of stress as a sign of the present younger generation's lack of stamina or 'character'. Having experienced the traumas of war, economic depression and the lack of any systematic provision for health care, it is hard for them to understand the perspective of our present 'have it all generation' in western society. More sinister predictions have been made by writers who feel that stress only represents individuals' lack of faith in community and lost sense of belonging. Where once hard work held meaning, by contrast, stress in the late twentieth century has contributed to a sense of *meaninglessness* (Sloan, 1996).

Jacobson has described the powerful 'professional mystique' which has arisen in what she calls the caring professions, saying that in searching for meaning, novelty and fulfilment in their work, carers look for – but do not always attain – certain expectations of caring work. Contrary to popular expectation, credentials do not always indicate competence or a high degree of success in work. Clients are not always co-operative and grateful, and professional status does not necessarily lead to personal autonomy and control over work. Perhaps most crushing of all is the realisation that relationships among professional colleagues are not all characteristically supportive or collegial (Jacobson & McGrath, 1983, p. 104).

The mismatch between the ideals of service and the value placed on the contributions of individual carers necessarily places a strain on the psychological and social contract between employers and employees, health care practitioners and their colleagues. It is not only the employees who suffer the consequences of the mismatch, however, as the sense of loss and insecurity evolves into feelings of 'stress' and burnout among staff whose patients and clients may receive substandard care as a result.

This takes us back to the discussion at the beginning of this chapter, when we looked at the ways in which people blame themselves for not coping with the challenges facing them, seeing it as a personal, rather than collective, failure to adapt to their particular circumstances. In trying to address the question of whether and why more strategic learning support systems are necessary to our ability to adapt to continuing personal and organisational change, we therefore need to begin closer to home, with an examination of the ways in which our feelings and beliefs about ourselves help us to maintain our sense of dignity and self-worth.

Why learning support is necessary

It will be argued here that learning support is needed to enable us to build relationships of value which will nurture and sustain us in our working and personal lives. At the most fundamental level we would argue that learning support is necessary:

- As a defence against feelings of disorientation, disillusionment and burn-out
- As a framework for clarifying our human values
- As a way to recover meaning in our social relationships
- As a means of providing skill rehearsal and of providing access to appropriate role models in the workplace (both personally and collegially)
- As a device for evaluating and disseminating best practice in health care
- As a way of acquiring 'emotional literacy' (i.e. the ability to deal constructively with our emotions in a mutually beneficial way).

A defence against disorientation, disillusionment and burn-out

Human defences against the effects of anxiety are well known to most health practitioners, who have been taught from day one of their careers that dealing with the public will require not only tact and sensitivity but also the need to distance oneself from human suffering in order to provide the best service to all patients. One way of illuminating and clarifying the moral, ethical and interpersonal problems associated with caring is the use of *narratives*.

In a treatise which examines the primacy of caring and the role of narratives in making sense of our experiences, Benner *et al.* (1996) explain that the practices and stories told within a given community provide some of the necessary background understanding for what they call 'ethical comportment' (p. 233). By sharing experiences, stories and concrete first-hand situations it is possible to formulate helpful narratives and 'memories of salient clinical situations' so that the transition from novice to skilful practitioner can be made (Benner *et al.*, 1996, p. 234).

In this way practice can be broken down and examined in its constituent parts so that the various fears, concerns, motivations and moral anxieties can be meaningfully addressed by practitioners. Such narratives can be presented in different ways according to the particular issues being discussed. For Benner *et al.*, working from a nursing ethos, there are two kinds of narratives, what the authors describe as 'constitutive and sustaining narratives' and 'narratives of learning'. Subtypes from these include narratives of healing, life-saving situations, stories which foster care and connection between patients and staff or patients and their loved ones, and stories of presencing or 'being there' for patients.

Constitutive or sustaining narratives 'depict situations that constitute the person's understanding of what it is to be a nurse' (Benner *et al.*, 1996, p. 237). For nurse we can of course directly substitute any kind of caring practitioner to the same effect. Such stories might help us to explore our beliefs and feelings about what it is to perform a particular role, and also to examine these as a way of producing a sense of shared understanding about the way we tackle situations and problems. The idea is presumably not only to examine potential issues of conflict and morality, but also to reward ourselves through recognition and affirmation for things we do right. Some cultures are more comfortable than others with praise; it may be that we have to learn to use praise constructively as part of our mutual defences against self-doubt and negativity. Such narratives can sustain us when things are not going so well.

Learning narratives are perhaps broader in their intent. They challenge us to be bold and to question our beliefs and practices to see where our judgements are flawed; to allow the possibility of learning to be contemplated by examining aspects of an issue which may not have occurred to us previously. Box 1.3 sets out the subthemes of learning narratives described by Benner *et al.* (1996, p. 237). Some readers may feel they have other narratives to add to these.

Box 1.3.

Learning the skill of involvement
Being open to experience
Narratives of disillusionment
Narratives of facing death and suffering
Liberation narratives

Any superficial glance at the daily newspapers, other media and the professional journals will pick up some of the narratives which could be described as narratives of disillusionment. The difference between what we expect and what we receive is easy to turn into a story with alternative perspectives playing the roles of victim or villain of the piece. Narratives of learning try to get under the skin of such accounts so that shortcomings are examined for their constituent parts. They are less concerned with exposing inadequacy and providing an opportunity to blame, and more concerned with acknowledging the constraints affecting practice both socially and bureaucratically.

The social sciences attempt to do this for us on a grander scale, with sociology exploring the structural and social antecedents to behaviour and effect within a given culture and psychology looking at the influence of attitudes and responses to determine the way we tackle human situations. At a much more personal and interpersonal level, learning narratives – particularly when supported by more experienced and understanding colleagues – are an excellent way to establish rapport and a sense of social and collegial support among professionals. Practitioners who take on active learning support roles can help to identify useful narratives of any kind which foster common understandings and which serve to remind us as professionals what we are here for.

The biggest problem facing practitioners who might be attracted to the notion of narratives is the immediate one of having sufficient physical resources (time and space) and the personal empathy and willingness necessary to do justice to such activities. Getting on with the job in hand is as much as many health professionals can face in the everyday hustle and bustle of caring work. What is needed is a practical and workable way of integrating such narratives into our everyday existence.

The temptation to make do and mend without any real contemplation of the bigger questions has a way of creeping up on carers of all disciplines and may be one reason why our personal health and well-being translate into the 'stress' narratives which are endemic in the literature. It is here that we have to turn to the literature on socialisation processes to see where we risk imbuing the wrong or inadequate kind of values to professionals at critical times of career transition.

Nothing is ever straightforward or clear-cut in human relationships and the narratives which have sustained different disciplines until now are not necessarily those that will sustain them in the future. It is important to bear this in mind before making any grand predictions for the good learning that support roles can achieve in professional practice.

The fact that a group of professionals adheres to one value system does not necessarily mean it is morally right either for them or their clients. Inter-professional working requires us to challenge the tribal practices and territorial claims of our own profession before going on to examine the cultural values of others. Then, and only then, can we begin to recognise each other's understandings for what they are: a cultural reproduction of what we experience daily in our working and professional lives. This brings us to the issue of *values* and what they mean for us socially.

A framework for clarifying human values

Values are implicit or explicit views about what we consider to be ideal. Values bring consistency to our behaviour and give us a sense of moral direction and personal and social identity (Kagan & Evans, 1995, pp. 12–13)

Problems at work emerge when our personal or collective values are challenged either by bureaucracy, by colleagues or by users of the service we provide. *Value systems* are those often unwritten values which together build a framework for understanding the norms of our experience. Values in health care usually concern the well-being of patients and clients and the ways in which we are expected to respond to their needs as well as their personal dignity and human rights.

Hafferty (1991) has described the process of *socialisation* to the workplace as a 'conscious strategy', a 'structure of norms about feelings and their management within the emergent subculture' experienced by practitioners. Hafferty is interested in the subculture of the medical school and the ways in which doctors and other health professionals create and maintain an emotional distance from the suffering of their patients. The values, behaviours and attitudes which doctors acquire can then be seen as a product of this process. Socialisation is thus a two-way process which shapes workers who go on to create social structures and systems guided by such values (Hafferty, 1991; Murphy, 1996).

Socialisation processes occur within organisations and work groups and are thought to help individuals recognise their roles and relative position in the organisational hierarchy. Socialisation could thus be described as 'the formal and informal social influence processes through which individuals acquire the skills, values and beliefs necessary for them to function as a member of the group or institution' (Nicholson, 1996, p. 167). *Professional socialisation* teaches workers at both a subliminal and conscious level which values are likely to bring them acceptance and reward within their chosen profession (Ewan & White, 1996).

Difficulties arise when our personal values clash with our professional values, or when the institutions in which we work get in the way of us behaving in accordance with those values. When the values we hold dear or consider important are challenged, we may react with defensiveness, aggression and a feeling of despondency (Kagan & Evans, 1995).

The resulting conflict between what we want to do and what we are made to do, because of constraints in the system, can cause a lot of misery and angst in both individuals and work groups and has been cited as one of the main sources of job dissatisfaction in health care work. Ewan and White have argued that we need to integrate values education more fully into the educational curriculum for health care. If we do not, we risk leaving practitioners to sort it out in the workplace where they are often under pressure and may not have the moral reasoning skills available to help them find acceptable solutions to ethical problems which arise. They describe socialisation as 'the hidden curriculum' which influences the judgement of students and which makes them aware of the informal and formal rules of participation in a given work culture (Ewan & White, 1996).

Additional problems can be created, however, when different value systems compete for attention. Value systems associated with medicine differ greatly between doctors and nurses, for example, with doctors being led by the biomedical, scientific paradigm (put crudely this *could* be seen as viewing patients as objects, as systems requiring repair and restoration via the wisdom of medical science) and nursing being viewed more as a caring and nurturing role where issues such as patient advocacy, emotional adjustment and adaptation to health and illness, and the importance of social context are emphasised in preference to physiological data and problems.

Different value systems of course reflect the education and training of professionals and the experiences through which they have learned to manage their roles in the health care hierarchy. Individuals may have trained in different settings, each of which have been exposed to different cultural norms and practices (consider for example the place of the family within different cultures) and at different times. The practice of separating sick and hospitalised children from their parents, for example, was considered valid and necessary to recuperation up until the late 1950s, a practice which contemporary thinking would view as cruel and psychologically damaging to both parents and child.

Practitioners of different generations and cultures can hold conflicting views about the appropriate way to behave in a given situation and their differences are unlikely to be resolved adequately unless some attempt is made to understand the thinking and value judgements behind their decisions. Some values may be acquired passively or intuitively, while others may need to be worked on to begin to make ethical sense to practitioners.

Trends in socialisation research are said to be moving away from 'the traditional view of the individual as a malleable recipient of influence towards a more active construction of individuals as agents of their own socialisation' (Nicholson, 1996, p. 168). Thus the impact of *formal socialisation processes* such as training, induction and supervision is thought to have less material effect on individual attitudes than those formal influences operating at the level of peer groups (Louis *et al.*, (1983) quoted in Nicholson, 1996, p. 168). Peer groups can therefore contribute significantly to the task of building a coherent value system.

Opportunities to build a values component into the health care education curriculum should therefore be accompanied by the conscious bringing together of different work groups in the workplace to see where values meet or diverge: to examine the core values they might share and to search out interprofessional solutions to the problems faced by practitioners. Learning support roles can help to do this by making the socialisation processes more explicit and providing both supporters and practitioners with legitimate opportunities for clarifying values and the ways in which competing value systems jostle for supremacy amid a host of other vested interests.

Helping practitioners to develop a viable alternative to the 'ethics of stoicism' which seems to prevail in health care (see Murphy, 1996) can in turn help us to value ourselves and others through active listening, respect for different world-views and an exploration of the different pressures and power structures which influence ethical decision-making in day-to-day practice.

The grindstone can be a very flinty place; everyone needs help now and then to clarify the issues bound up in everyday moral dilemmas (which often come in puzzling disguises) and to be able to argue and defend different positions in relation to individual parties without resorting to rivalries and power games and the imposition of one value system above all others.

A way to recover meaning in social relationships

One of our first concerns must be to know what constitutes meaning in human experience. For some, it is the feelings, intentions, hopes, sensed expectations and desires of people which constitute the 'lifeworlds' we all inhabit (Sloan, 1996; Habermas, 1979).

The ways in which we develop and build meaning are affected by the relationships we make (or have foisted on us) at work, by bureaucracy or in our personal lives. Meanings then constitute our environment for each other (Marris, 1996, p. 79). Meanings are constantly manipulated in our interactions with each other and in the decisions made on our behalf by policymakers and our public institutions. Even where we may share common meanings – for example, being a parent or a friend – what the experience of being a parent or friend *means* will still be unique to each of us depending on differences of culture, upbringing, socialisation, education and expectation.

It would seem that from an early age we become quite adept at juggling these different kinds of meaning every day as we constantly adapt to changes in our environment and others' expectations of us. The meanings attached to roles and relationships at work are a way of helping us to shift gear, to adapt to changing circumstances, and when they are effective then the process of adaptation and learning may be less painful than if roles were unclear or our relationships confused.

Meanings are of course open to multiple and conflicting interpretations and may or may not be shared. This, we would argue, is the root of the difficulty health professionals experience in their attempts to reconcile expectations of themselves and their personal contribution to those with other diverse agendas. A social worker's understanding of a patient's most acute problems will no doubt differ from those expressed by the patient's physician, dietitian or physiotherapist.

A junior doctor's perception of need may well focus on the immediate tasks required to take an accurate medical history and formulate a reliable diagnosis, rather than the long-term focus of what disability may mean for patients and their families.

And while we clearly do not have time for the luxury of sharing all the perceptions and meanings we bring to a clinical situation, we could benefit from a closer examination and understanding of some of the key issues. Misunderstandings concerning another member of the health care team can sometimes result purely from a misinterpretation (or ignorance of) the professional or personal demands being made on that person at a given moment. All too often another person's agenda is assumed, rather than made explicit, so that barriers between professionals build without any attempt to explore the issues behind them.

Explanations of meaning can help us to clarify what is important to us in terms of immediate needs and long-term values, and can help us to define and communicate roles more easily, to discover where the interpersonal and structural boundaries lie, and to bring into focus those areas where our interpretations or world-views may diverge from others so that the search for shared meanings can begin.

The search for shared meaning

In exploring further the nature of meaning in relation to our psychological attachment to each other, Marris suggests that meanings can be divided into three areas or realms: personal, mutual and public meanings.

Personal meanings occur at the most fundamental level of human experience and come from the experience of attachment:

> 'They organise the concerns which underlie our search for relationships, our defences, denials and strategies of control. They underlie what others perceive as our character or personality.'

> (Marris, 1996, p. 79)

Mutual meaning is represented in the common language of interaction. This enables us to negotiate, describe and clarify what we intend or infer by our actions and intentions, to define mutual expectations, to reflect on situations and to clarify and affirm or deny mutual understandings of what we mean:

> 'Mutual meanings also articulate what is happening, why it matters and what is to be done, but in terms now that enable each to make their intentions, responses, feelings intelligible to the other.'

> (Marris, 1996, p. 80)

Public Meanings help us to organise our experience into recognisable entities, for example, concerning ideas of family, organisational structures and 'rules' which define our existence for us. Large scale examples of this might be in systems of taxation, education or the criminal justice system of a given society. For Marris such systems:

> 'are authoritative, because we recognise and feel compelled by the logic of structures whose rules and assumptions we accept. The assumptions which define a community of discourse of which we are part have, then, the power to determine for us, irrespective of our wishes, meanings we *have* to acknowledge.' [emphasis added]

> (Marris, 1996, p. 81)

Meanings are thus constantly responded to, challenged, renegotiated, re-evaluated, trusted by some and abhorred by others. Our interpretation of meaning at the personal, mutual and public levels therefore helps to shape our common understanding of a situation and gives us the opportunity to refine and develop our understandings as we engage with others in a process of mutual negotiation.

Learning support which is theoretically sound and which has the confidence of both employers and employees can therefore help us to establish, through negotiation, where our problems come from and where a divergence of opinion or expectation can lead to disappointment, disillusionment or plain old misunderstanding of each other's meanings and values. Unfortunately, this is easier to say than achieve. Before we can succeed in sharing meanings it is important to take a critical look at some of the meanings – or in this case assumptions – regarding the standards health professionals are expected to live up to. A useful starting point might be to evaluate from our own perspectives some of the political and professional *rhetoric* which infuses our working lives.

The politics of rhetoric

The word 'rhetoric' refers here to the language and concepts employed to persuade and influence people. Rhetorics help to highlight the assumptions and values which underpin our actions and motivations; hence an examination of rhetoric can help us to account for what we do and why we do it in a particular way.

The particular *political rhetorics* that will come under scrutiny here are the rhetorics of:

- 'Professional accountability'
- 'Lifelong learning' and 'the learning society'
- 'Reflective practice'.

Health professionals can feel discomfort when the rhetorics or ideals they are expected to live up to are beyond both their resources and their autonomy to provide. This is the case regardless of whether you are the chief executive of a health care provider or the person managing the catering contract. Concerns over whether you have the money, supplies, personnel and skills available to meet the standards required affect all providers. A Mr Micawber shortfall between budget and expenditure has implications for all aspects of the service, regardless of the provider's perceived 'place' in the organisational hierarchy.

When the discomfort becomes too great, people experiencing it can react in very different ways. Some may express outward compliance but feel inward dejection and protect themselves by distancing themselves psychologically (i.e. 'it's only work'). They may vote with their feet and choose a less problematic way of earning a living, hence the recurring recruitment and retention problems experienced by health care employers. Alternatively, they may internalise their worries, perceiving themselves as somehow failing to make the grade expected of them. For a few, the discomfort arouses feelings of injustice and anger which may spur them on to challenge the status quo, and it is the person who challenges the system who can then be perceived as the troublemaker or outsider who tries to 'rock the boat'.

At one time the people with the specialist skills were the most successful at rocking boats. At the inception of the NHS in Britain, for example, consultant physicians and public health officials ruled the roost in deciding on post-war national priorities and large scale public health programmes. The mystique surrounding medical knowledge helped to concentrate power among doctors. During the twentieth century medicine became integral to the social and political apparatus of industrialised societies (Porter, 1997, p. 666).

There are some who believe that medicine has acquired too much power, however, and there is evidence of 'a growing movement directed towards encouraging patient assertiveness [and this] is accepted as a sign of a diminishing of medical dominance' in health care (Lupton, 1994, p. 113). This challenge to the professional dominance of medicine has also been engineered by central governments who attempt to put the rhetoric of 'quality' to work within a framework of professional accountability, so that complex systems and dynamics of consumer charters, league tables, codes of professional practice and benchmarks are designed to try and encourage compliance to certain expectations, and to attempt to protect the public from poor performance on the part of professional care providers. The end result is that all practitioners feel under pressure to deliver to this standard.

In the UK the medical profession in particular has been under intense pressure to formulate stricter self-regulation practices following concerns that doctors are not sufficiently accountable for their decisions and practice. The fear for them has been that if a satisfactory system of self-regulation is not imposed, then an independent regulatory body (with all the political connotations that that implies) will be set up to protect the public from unsafe practice. 'This move marks a milestone in the regulation of doctors' (Laurance, 1999).

The methods of self-regulation employed may not meet with the approval of a profession which has by practice and tradition set its own professional agenda. There are also concerns that any system of imposed regulation will be difficult to manage and monitor appropriately, a situation which teachers and other educationists have already experienced through the workings of the Office for Standards in Education (OFSTED). The resulting damage to the morale of staff who fail to comply or meet with expected standards has serious implications for future recruitment and retention of staff, even if the policy of regulation succeeds in giving the public greater confidence in the services of the public sector. The philosopher Michel Foucault might have seen this as a 'swarming of disciplinary mechanisms' exercised by government in an attempt to control an otherwise powerful sector of society (Foucault, 1977 (translated by Sheridan) p. 211).

The membership of particular professional groups thus implies the need to understand and adhere to the standards required (both politically and pragmatically) of that professional group. Such rhetorics are of course not exclusive to health care but can be found in any workplace, rooted as they are in broader governmental drives towards the global rhetoric of cost-effectiveness and economic competitiveness.

Professional accountability is therefore inextricably linked to economic concerns regarding the financial sustainability of populations, and each profession has to devise its own way of responding to the demands made on it by its own ethical appraisal of the decisions and choices made by that profession on the public's behalf.

Overshadowing all care provision is the legacy twenty-first century medicine must carry into the future. The historian Roy Porter, in closing his monumental account of what benefits medicine has brought to humanity, expresses the moral dilemmas faced by skilled practitioners in a world with an unlimited propensity for disease and want:

> 'The close of my history thus suggests that medicine's finest hour is the dawn of its dilemmas. For centuries medicine was impotent and unproblematic. From the Greeks to the First World War, its tasks were simple: to grapple with lethal diseases and gross disabilities, to ensure live births and manage pain. It performed these with meagre success. Today, with 'mission accomplished', its triumphs are dissolving in disorientation. Medicine has led to inflated expectations, which the public easily swallowed. Yet as those expectations become unlimited, they are unfulfillable: medicine will have to redefine its limits even as it extends its capacities.'

> (Porter, 1997, p. 718)

As old, inherited power structures crumble, everyone involved in health care will feel the effects. Mass disorientation and inflated, unfulfillable expectations are the context in which professional accountabilities must evolve themselves in the world's wealthier economies. The rhetoric of professional accountability cannot therefore be reduced to simple codes of conduct or practice, but must rather seek to establish itself as a way of constructing and effecting meaning for those of us who are trying to grapple with the 'unfulfillable' demands made on us. The practice of accountability requires us to recognise and acknowledge the limits of our competence as individuals, and the provision of learning support in particular is seen as one way of allowing practitioners to rehearse their own professional judgements and limits to practice.

Practitioners who take on formal support roles have a vital part to play in establishing and maintaining the right conditions in the workplace for the enactment of appropriate skills and attitudes. The chapters which follow will critically assess the pivotal role of mentors, preceptors and clinical supervisors in bringing about these conditions, and will examine the tools and attributes they use to do this in clinical situations.

The rhetoric of 'lifelong learning' and the 'learning society'

One of the ways of responding to the burgeoning demand on practitioners has been to try and inculcate the professional ethos with the capacity for 'lifelong learning'. As medicine and information technology advance, we are faced with increasing technical (and technocratic) specialisation, and the fragmentation of old certainties into new, information over-loaded specialisms requiring ever more sophisticated knowledge to manage them. It has been argued that the utilitarian, socio-economic rationale of training to carry out a specific function, or education to minimum standards for future employment, is giving way to a more holistic and visionary view of education as a lifelong process:

> 'The old industrial society model of education, which tends to fragment and narrow it into predetermined patterns and outcomes, is changing to the information society model, which educates for a wider and more responsible role in a democratic society.'

> (Longworth & Davies, 1996, p. 9)

The rhetoric devised to manage the information society model finds expression in many of the concepts introduced into the workplace and educational institutions over the past 50 years. *Learning* as a *lifelong process* is now seen to be part of the strategic investment society must make for promoting the economic and social well-being of nations (Tuijnman, 1996, p. 36). The related idea of a *learning society* assumes that certain types of social arrangements are more likely to promote lifelong learning than others, although specific studies of learning within social institutions have rarely been accompanied by a wider conceptual framework on what we mean by societal learning (Schuller & Field, 1998, p. 226).

When we expect social groups (as part of wider society) to learn, therefore, we have to be careful not to assume simply that they will have the willingness or wherewithal to do so on their own. Armstrong, for example, has argued that the idea of a learning society is really only a veneer, 'glossing over fundamental political and cultural differences that are no longer exposed for critical examination' (Armstrong, 1998, p. 4). Does the concept of a learning society exist only to advance certain political ideological ends, for example, or is it a genuine attempt to see that every community takes steps to ensure its members have the different kinds of knowledge considered necessary for life? (See Hughes & Tight, 1995; van der Zee, 1996). Armstrong argues that the concept of a 'learning society' is in reality a rhetorical construct which has not been sufficiently challenged for its value to society.

Some of the critical questions which might be aimed at the concept include those concerning social capital generally. *Social capital* refers to the level of trust which exists in the social environment and the extent to which mutual obligations between people are upheld (Schuller & Field, 1998, p. 226). The questions we may want to ask ourselves as professionals concern very pragmatic issues at both the personal and mutual level of meaning. For example, what are the kinds of context and culture which promote communication and mutual learning as part of the fabric of everyday life? And what kinds of institutional relationship are most supportive of learning in social life? (Schuller & Field, 1998, p. 234).

Nolan *et al.* (1999, p. 5) have warned that underlying the current rhetoric of lifelong learning there is the potential for conflict, particularly regarding equity of access and opportunities:

- 'Between education as a guardian of values and as a vehicle for economic prosperity
- Between the aspirations of individuals and the aims of large corporate bodies
- In balancing responsibilities for paying for lifelong learning and ensuring that certain sections of the population are not further disadvantaged.'

We need to take care, then, that when we are asked to participate in developing the *'learning society'*, the *'learning organisation'* or indeed the *'learning company'*, we do not inadvertently swallow the rhetoric of lifelong learning without due consideration of the demands such participation requires of individuals and institutions.

The proliferation of learning opportunities in health care education in recent years to fulfil the onus on us to be sufficiently 'updated' and therefore responsible lifelong learners, has placed increasing budgetary as well as time constraints on professionals (THES, 1999). While many professionals have responded to this challenge with enthusiasm and interest, we have to take care to see that the very act of *formal learning* does not prohibit other creative ways of bringing social capital – and therefore, trust – into the workplace. The opportunities which come from informal learning are not necessarily recognised through formal 'certificates' and credentialling, but they nevertheless have an important role to play in making learning accessible to greater numbers of people. Such opportunities are under-researched in the literature on adult learning. In particular, the relationships between family, work and adult life need to be made more explicit so that education and training policies can more accurately reflect the needs and motivations of learners (Blaxter *et al.*, 1997, p. 137).

Lifelong learning, and the means to achieve it, are not understood in the same way by all learners and learning communities and this needs to be recognised if we are to increase workplace learning opportunities in the future.

The rhetoric of 'reflective practice'

The focus on practice and the incorporation of reflection as a learning tool in workplace education is thought to enable learners to solve problems in practice. By exploring their unique situations, learners may be encouraged to generate new knowledge (Schon, 1991; Murphy & Atkins, 1994).

Schon has pointed to the limitations of the 'technical-rationality' model of professional education, and to the 'crisis of legitimacy' rooted in the perceived failure of professionals to live up to their own and society's expectations as a consequence of their dependence on the status of the scientific method. In his view, we have increasingly become aware of the importance to actual practice of various phenomena: of complexity, uncertainty, instability, uniqueness and value-conflict, none of which readily fit the model of technical rationality he describes.

Problem-*solving* is in itself not enough to teach us what it is to be competent or professional, rather:

> 'In real world practice, problems do not present themselves to the practitioner as givens. They must be constructed from the materials of problematic situations which are puzzling, troubling and uncertain. In order to convert a problematic situation to a problem, a practitioner must do a certain kind of work. He must make sense of an uncertain situation that initially makes no sense.'

> (Schon, 1991, p. 40)

The difficulty for health care is that unlike the 'high hard ground' described by Schon as the place where practitioners can make effective use of research-based theory, health care is emotion-laden and practice settings tend to resemble his 'swampy lowlands', where situations appear to be confusing 'messes' incapable of technical solution (Schon, 1991, p. 42).

The skills of reflection on and in practice have been hailed as the holy grail for nurses and other health care staff as a way of helping to make messy, swampy, puzzling situations clearer. The move away from traditional positivistic and behaviourist paradigms towards more emancipatory curricula in nursing education has given reflection an important role as an:

> 'appropriate vehicle for the analysis of nursing practice, fostering not only an understanding of nurses' work, but also the development of the critically thoughtful approaches essential for providing nursing care in complex environments.'
>
> (Pierson, 1998, p. 165)

The growth and interest in the conception of reflection has been felt in a wide range of literature and practices across the field of lifelong learning generally (Edwards, 1997, p. 152). It is important to be aware, however, that as with all forms of teaching and pedagogy, every method has its limitations, and some of these are already beginning to be expressed in the literature.

Dependence on reflective journals, diaries, portfolios, critical incident analyses and role play has led to reflection being seen as the answer to many of the prayers of those involved in health care education, for a method which will help practitioners to analyse their own behaviours as well as the problems patients bring to them.

Edwards has warned, however, that reflection is not a neutral process in professional practice. It can serve a range of interests and have a variety of ambivalent and contradictory consequences. Reflective practice does not in itself guarantee neutrality, nor can it be seen as a universal description of professional practice and professional identity. Instead, it may be yet another form of 'moral technology' and a form of governmentality through which professional work is intensified and indeed regulated/made accountable (Edwards, 1997, p. 153).

Where reflection is used to promote the personal growth or development of the practitioner it is constrained by many factors, including the time and support available to make it relevant to employees or students, the limits on privacy, comfort with self-disclosure and the ability to provide an atmosphere of trust and collegiality in which individuals can express themselves openly and honestly (Landeen *et al.*, 1992, p. 354).

When examining the claims made for reflective practice, then, we need to be sensitive to the conditions which inhibit or promote helpful learning situations, otherwise we stand to lose the trust of practitioners who place their faith in these methods as a way of helping them to become competent and caring. There is a need to be alert to the emotional labour involved in caring for others (Staden, 1998) and to respect the individual's rights to confidentiality in a learning situation.

The exploration of rhetorics such as these therefore allows us to see the dangers of some of the assumptions underlying common practices in health care, and stresses the importance of shared meaning in our interactions with others. The pragmatics of providing skill rehearsal and access to appropriate role models in the workplace via learning support are therefore a logical place to move on to in the context of health care work.

A means of providing skill rehearsal and access to appropriate role models

Mentoring, preceptorship and clinical supervision are relatively recent innovations in health care work. Bond and Holland probably speak for a lot of practitioners when they describe the problems associated with the introduction of yet more changes in management practice (in their case, they are referring to the introduction of clinical supervision in nursing):

> 'As with all holy grails, it attracts both devotees and non-believers and it is the search that can often attract the most attention and noise. Many pilgrims flock to support it, some out of genuine belief, some because it's the fashionable thing to do. Many may pay lip service to the creed but, either wittingly, or unwittingly, will be highly selective or shallow in putting it into everyday practice. Many will view it simply as the unearthing of old relics and scriptures which they had problems worshipping the first time around...'

(Bond & Holland, 1998, p. 2)

Following fashion in health care is hard to avoid, particularly as wave upon wave of paper and policy continue to swamp us in the workplace. First there are strategic national policies to do with management, education and policy, and then there are the professional, technical and legal ramifications of policies which need to be attended to in quick succession. The provision of learning support which attempts to help practitioners implement policy at a local and practical level therefore has to be responsive to fluid and ever changing scenarios and directions.

Skills, or the lack of them, are a continuing concern for health care employers, and the problems of developing and maintaining an adequate human resource to manage increasing workloads constitute a colossal managerial and educational challenge. Learning support has the potential to provide concrete opportunities for learning at the level of peer groups, as an educational strategy between the experienced and inexperienced employee, and as a way of giving employees access to informed guidance and moral support as a basis on which to build appropriate career decisions.

Although clinical supervision has a distinguished history in psychiatry and social work, mentoring has largely been developed in business and industry, while preceptorship has become more widely accepted as a valuable means of assisting the newly qualified (or new in post) in their transition from student to qualified practitioner. The literatures on all three have developed fairly arbitrarily, however, with no one method appearing to offer the complete solution to problems experienced by the professions.

In the chapters which follow the relationships and boundaries between each of these support roles will be debated and clarified. Since the publication of the first edition of this book in 1993, we, as authors, have had the benefit of engaging in empirical and practice-based research which has allowed us to develop our theories in action, i.e. the evidence base for our theories and suppositions about learning support has been widely challenged, so that the claims we make for such support are now firmly grounded in actual practice as experienced by practitioners of many professional hues.

This does not mean that we have the definitive answers to the problems that practitioners face, but it does mean that the models of learning support we have devised, and which will be outlined in detail in Chapters 2, 3 and 4, have a solid base in real-world practice. The evidence we offer here has been subject to peer review in the workplace, and subject to the scrutiny of pilgrims and cynics alike. We have not attempted to chocolate-coat or gild the experiences we have encountered in our own holy grail for the perfect support networks, but would rather wish to engage readers in a critical reappraisal of what support systems can do to enhance the experience of practitioners, and we hope the care of patients and clients as an adjunct. This requires us to assess the value of learning support as a potential mechanism for communicating best practice through the constant re-evaluation and dissemination of 'best practice' in health care.

A device for evaluating and disseminating best practice in health care

We must first add a caveat. Learning support does not *automatically* lead to best practice in respect of care interventions. No system which depends on human beings for its existence could hope to ensure that best practice was attainable all the time. Rather, learning support attempts to create and maintain the required atmosphere of collegiality and trust which can help practitioners to challenge those areas of practice or intervention which have so far failed to respond adequately to the needs of patients and clients. Learning support alone cannot turn beginners into experts; that is a task for education, experience and practitioners themselves. What it can do is help practitioners to articulate their discomforts and uncertainties, admit to their lack of knowledge without fear of being seen as weak or helpless, and devise ways of overcoming the constraints on acquiring a sense of confidence and self-esteem, which so often seem to characterise the pressures on health care staff (see Stoter (1997) for example).

Individuals have different ways of expressing their sense of vulnerability and cannot always find the courage to do this (even to themselves). In our brave new world of high technology institutional health care and the constrained old world of care within the community, best practice can only be achieved when practitioners have a grasp of the unevenness and confusion of human needs and coping strategies. The 'dawning of medicine's dilemmas' (see Porter (1997), p. 718) is the necessary realisation that what constitutes best practice for one person may not be seen as such by another. Needs and care are culturally relative; they cannot be set in stone, and even where evidence is research based, what helps one person does not necessarily help another. For the new recruit who is eager to put the world to rights, or the employee who began work when traditional hierarchies seemed to hold more sway, this can be a deeply disturbing and distressing discovery.

The lack of moral certainties requires imaginative and reflexive ways of looking at the world, and effective support at critical times of career transition can make this process more attainable than if the employee remains unsupported and under the misapprehension that someone, somewhere is going to show him or her where those wished-for certainties lie.

All of which brings us to another important function for learning support. Perhaps the strongest of all arguments for learning support provision lies in the need for practitioners to acquire personal strategies which will help them to survive emotionally in practice situations. The neglect of the emotional component of caring and health care work has led to much heartache for practitioners, and just as the literature has begun to appreciate the need to help individuals balance the emotional with their professional lives, so too do we wish to consider the impact of emotions on practitioners' well-being and sense of self.

A way of acquiring emotional literacy

Managing stage fright in the theatre of life is how one author describes the geography of emotions and emotional relationships in social life (Freund, 1998, pp. 268–9). Freund builds on the seminal work of Goffman (1959) by exploring the nature of self as a social actor. Just how do we sustain performances, maintain appearances and protect personal and team secrets, when exposed to the very public domains of our working lives? How do we keep up the pretences of caring when we know we are just too tired, too befuddled or too overworked to cope?

What emotions does health work generate, and is it acceptable to express these emotions in our interactions at work? Most professionals have acquired the ability to temper real feelings with a public face. As Nicky James has explained in her account of emotional labour and cancer, the phrase *emotional labour* is intended to highlight similarities as well as differences between emotional and physical labour:

> 'with both being hard, skilled work requiring experience, affected by immediate conditions, external controls and subject to divisions of labour.'

> (James, 1993, p. 95)

Arlie Hochschild, the author most identified with the concept of emotional labour, has criticised the lack of grounded, highly nuanced studies that allow us to piece together a coherent portrait of emotion in organisations (Hochschild, 1993, p. xii). Social psychologists are berated for their willingness to study organisations and issues such as worker satisfaction, while treating emotions as marginal, rather than central to life at work. And while it is certainly the case that emotions have come to be taken more seriously as a psychological health issue, few people have the opportunity to undergo structured educational programmes on the management of emotions, or on the acquisition of emotional literacy or intelligence (see Goleman, 1995; Weisinger, 1998).

The acceptance of emotion work as critical to caring is increasing, but for those health professionals who hold dear to the scientific rationale of health care, emotionality can seem a frightening and perhaps unnecessary diversion from otherwise important and more rational conceptions of work. The old adage of keeping one's professional or emotional distance from the gritty realities of human experience has a long and venerated position in the psychology of health care, and not necessarily just in western cultures. Explanations for this vary, with some blame being laid at the door of gender stereotyping and the side-lining of emotions as women's domain (Duncombe & Marsden, 1998). Disagreements about gender differences have tended to polarise arguments and site discussions about gender in the feminist literature, without adequate attention being paid to the centrality of emotions to human experience. It may be that it is not only people who feel, but organisations too (Albrow, 1997), and that cultural studies in organizations need to focus more directly on this important phenomenon (Putnam & Mumby, 1993).

We would argue that on the basis of our experience of providing learning support, the development of a language which helps people to become more emotionally literate is an important if not core function of support roles in the workplace. *Emotional literacy* is as vital to human communication as speech and hearing. If we fail to develop it, and depend on other instincts to defend us and help us to deal with our anxieties, then we risk reaping the consequences of our illiteracy, which is the breakdown of communication and the sense of personal failure and being overwhelmed which may permeate our working lives.

Policies which address workplace problems such as bullying, aggression, violence in the workplace, emotional stress and feelings of helplessness, fail to recognise one vital component of managing emotional responses. In order to manage the emotions of others, it is necessary to recognise and manage the emotions we experience ourselves. Emotional responses rarely reflect only one side of an argument. Without this important dimension we may not succeed in giving the right signals or responses to those we communicate with; we may not appreciate the subtleties of what we say and do in our interactions with others, and above all we may not be able to respect the opinions of others without the feeling of having our points of view respected in kind. By utilising learning support to develop greater emotional awareness, it is sometimes possible to circumvent some of the ill feeling which is cogently expressed in a treatise on the emotional cost of health care work and nursing in particular:

> '... Overworked, underpaid and undervalued; the trinity of nursing misery is related with depressing regularity ... Years of uninterrupted nursing is bad for your emotional health. Human beings have a basic need to be around healthy, happy people ... No other caring profession expects its members to soldier on until they drop.'

> (Munro, 1999, p. 15)

And while we do not advocate soldiering on as a strategy for health care work, either, we do feel the need for nurses and other health professionals to take emotional charge of their futures by challenging the status quo. They are not alone in feeling the way they do, and interprofessional collaboration on the ways in which learning support can help us to articulate our frustrations more positively is in our view a useful beginning and a starting point for considering new ways of thinking and acting.

References

Albrow, M. (1997) *Do Organizations Have Feelings?* Routledge, London.

Armstrong, P. (1998) Rhetoric and reification: disconnecting research, teaching, and learning in the learning society. *Proceedings of the 28th Annual Scutrea Conference*, University of Exeter, pp. 4–15.

Barber, P. (1996) Social symbolism of health: the notion of the soul in professional care. In: *Sociology: Insights in Health Care*, (ed. A. Perry), pp. 54–82. Edward Arnold, London.

Benner, P.A., Tanner, C.A. & Chesla, C.A. (1996) *Expertise in Nursing Practice – Caring, Clinical Judgment and Ethics*, Springer Publishing Company, New York.

Blaxter, L., Hughes,C. & Tight, M. (1997) Education, work and adult life: how adults relate their learning to their work, family and social lives. In: *Adult Learning, A Reader*, (P. Sutherland), pp. 135–147. Kogan Page, London.

Bond, M. & Holland, S. (1998) *Skills of Clinical Supervision for Nurses*, Open University Press, Buckingham.

Borrill, C.S., Wall, T.D. & West, M.A. (1996) *Mental Health of the NHS Workforce*. Institute of Work Psychology, University of Sheffield and Department of Psychology, University of Leeds.

Borrill, C.S., Wall, T.D., West, M.A., Hardy, G.E., Shapiro, D.A., Haynes, C.E., Stride,C.B., Woods, D. & Carter, A.J. (1998) *Stress among staff in NHS Trusts*. Final Report, Institute of Work Psychology, University of Sheffield and Psychological Therapies Research Centre, University of Leeds.

Brookfield, S.D. (1987) *Developing Critical Thinkers: Challenging Adults to Explore New Ways of Thinking and Acting.* Jossey-Bass, San Francisco.

Davies, C. (1995) *Gender and the Professional Predicament in Nursing.* Open University Press, Buckingham.

Duncombe, J. & Marsden, D. (1998) 'Stepford wives' and 'hollow men'? Doing emotion work, doing gender and 'authenticity' in intimate heterosexual relationships. In: *Emotions and Social Life – Critical Themes and Contemporary Issues*, (eds G. Bendelow & S.J. Williams), pp. 211–27. Routledge, London.

Edwards, R. (1997) *Changing Places? Flexibility, Lifelong Learning and a Learning Society.* Routledge, London.

Eraut, M. (1994) *Developing Professional Knowledge and Competence.* Falmer Press, London.

Ewan, C. & White, R. (1996) *Teaching Nursing – a Self-Instructional Handbook*, 2nd edn. Chapman & Hall, London.

Foucault, M. (1977) (Translated by Sheridan) *Discipline and Punish – the Birth of the Prison.* Penguin, London.

Freund, P.E.S. (1998) Social performances and their discontents – the biopsychosocial aspects of dramaturgical stress. In: *Emotions and Social Life – Critical Themes and Contemporary Issues*, (eds G. Bendelow & S. J. Williams), pp. 268–94. Routledge, London.

Fukuyama, F. (1996) *Trust – the Social Virtues and the Creation of Prosperity.* Free Press Paperbacks, New York.

Goffman, E. (1959) *The Presentation of Self in Everyday Life.* Doubleday Anchor, New York.

Goleman, D. (1995) *Emotional Intelligence.* Bantam, New York.

Good, B.J. (1994) *Medicine, Rationality and Experience: an Anthropological Perspective.* Cambridge University Press, Cambridge.

Habermas, J. (1979) *Communication and the Evolution of Society.* Beacon Press, Boston.

Hafferty, F.W. (1991) *Into the Valley: Death and the Socialization of Medical Students.* Yale University Press, Newhaven.

Hart, M.U. (1992) *Working and Educating for Life.* Routledge, London.

Herriot, P., Hirsh,W. & Reilly, P. (1998) *Trust and Transition: Managing Today's Employment Relationship.* John Wiley & Sons, Chichester.

Hochschild, A. (1993) Preface. In: *Emotion in Organizations, (ed. S. Fineman).* Sage, London.

Holden, R.J. (1991) An analysis of caring: attributions, contributions and resolutions. *Journal of Advanced Nursing,* **16**, 893–8.

Holland, J.W. (1995) *A Doctor's Dilemma – Stress and the Role of the Carer.* Free Association Books, London.

Hughes, C. & Tight, M. (1995) The myth of the learning society. *British Journal of Educational Studies,* **43** (3), 290–304.

Jacobson, S.F. & McGrath, H.M. (1983) *Nurses Under Stress,* Wiley, New York.

James, N. (1993) Divisions of emotional labour: disclosure and cancer. In: *Emotion in Organizations,* (ed. S. Fineman), pp. 94–117. Sage, London.

Kagan, C. & Evans, J. (1995) *Professional Interpersonal Skills for Nurses.* Chapman & Hall, London.

Landeen, J., Byrne, C. & Brown, B. (1992) Journal keeping as an educational strategy in teaching psychiatric nursing. *Journal of Advanced Nursing,* **17**, 347–55.

Laurance, J. (1999) Skills tests for doctors. *The Independent,* 11 February.

Longworth, N. & Davies, K.W. (1996) *Lifelong Learning: New Vision, New Implications, New Roles for People, Organizations, Nations and Communities in the 21st Century.* Kogan Page, London.

Louis, M.R., Posner, P.Z. & Powell, G.N. (1983) The availability and helpfulness of socialisation practices. *Personnel Psychology,* **36**, 857–66.

Lupton, D. (1994) *Medicine as Culture: Illness, Disease and the Body in Western Culture.* Sage, London.

Marris, P. (1996) *The Politics of Uncertainty – Attachment in Private and Public Life.* Routledge, London.

Munro, R. (1999) Consider the emotional cost of nursing, (Sideview). *Nursing Times,* **95** (6), 15.

Murphy, J. (1996) *Using Health & Illness to Understand Social Psychological Problems and Perspectives.* The Open University, Milton Keynes.

Murphy, K. & Atkins, S. (1994) Reflection within a practice led curriculum. In: *Reflective Practice in Nursing: the Growth of the Professional Practitioner,* (eds A. Palmer, S. Burns & C. Bulman), pp. 10–17. Blackwell Science, Oxford.

Nicholson, N. (1996) Careers in a new context. In: *Psychology at Work,* (ed. P. Warr), pp. 161–87. Penguin, London.

Nolan, M. Owen R. & Venables, A. (1999) Conflicts in continuing education, *Nursing Times Learning Curve*, **3** (1), 3 March, 5–6.

Perry, A. (1993) A sociologist's view: the handmaiden's theory. In: *Nursing – Its Hidden Agendas*, (eds M. Jolley & G. Brykczynska), pp. 43–79. Edward Arnold, London.

Pierson, W. (1998) Reflection and Nursing Education. *Journal of Advanced Nursing*, **27**, 165–70.

Porter, R. (1997) *The Greatest Benefit to Mankind: a Medical History of Humanity from Antiquity to the Present.* Harper Collins, London.

Putnam, L.L. & Mumby, D.K. (1993) *Organizations, emotions and the myth of rationality.* In: *Emotion in Organizations*, (ed. S. Fineman), pp. 36–57. Sage, London.

Rogers, R. Salvage, J. & Cowell, R. (1999) *Nurses at Risk – a Guide to Health & Safety at Work*, 2nd edn. Macmillan Press Ltd, Basingstoke.

Schon, D. (1991) *The Reflective Practitioner – How Professionals Think in Action.* Arena, London.

Schuller, T. & Field, J. (1998) Social Capital, Human Capital and the Learning Society. *International Journal of Lifelong Education*, **17**, (4), 226–35.

Sennett, R. (1998) *The Corrosion of Character – Personal Consequences of Work in the New Capitalism.* W.W. Norton & Co, New York.

Sloan, T. (1996) *Damaged Life: the Crisis of the Modern Psyche.* Routledge, London.

Staden, H. (1998) Alertness to the needs of others: a study of the emotional labour of caring. *Journal of Advanced Nursing*, **27**, 147–56.

Stoter, D. (1997) *Staff Support in Health Care.* Blackwell Science, Oxford.

Teasdale, K.(1998) *Advocacy in Health Care.* Blackwell Science, Oxford.

THES (1999) Why I believe lifelong learning is making nurses leave the NHS, (J. Hewison). Soapbox, *Times Higher Education Supplement*, 22 January, p.18.

Tschudin, V. (1997) The emotional cost of caring. In: *Caring: the Compassion and Wisdom of Nursing*, (ed. G. Brykczynska), pp. 157–179. Edward Arnold, London.

Tuijnman, A.C. (1996) The expansion of adult education and training in Europe: trends and issues. In: *The Learning Society: Challenges and Trends*, (eds P. Raggatt, R. Edwards & N. Small), pp. 26–44. Routledge, London.

Weisinger, H. (1998) *Emotional Intelligence at Work – the Untapped Edge for Success.* Jossey-Bass, San Francisco.

van der Zee, H. (1996) The learning society. In: *The Learning Society: Challenges and Trends*, (eds P. Raggatt, R. Edwards & N. Small), pp. 162–83.

Chapter 2
Mentoring in Practice

'Come to the edge', he said.
They said, 'We are afraid'.
'Come to the edge', he said.
They came.
He pushed them ...
and they flew!

Giullaume Apollinaire

Introduction

The complex, intriguing concept of mentoring continues to tax authors and researchers from a variety of different disciplines as they explore the role of mentors in a range of settings that includes the health, education and business arenas. From its origins in classical Greece through business interpretations of the 1970s with adaptations in education and nursing during the 1980s, much has been written about the subject and a multitude of different approaches taken (Merriam, 1993; Fish, 1995; Weightman, 1996; Jarvis & Gibson, 1997).

Mentoring has become a high profile topic in business, women's magazines, the press and nursing, and it is beginning to find its place in current teacher preparation, the police service and the medical profession (Smith & West-Burnham, 1993; Tomlinson, 1995; Freeman, 1997). Mentoring has associations with the personal and professional development of individuals in a wide variety of organisational settings. It is also seen as a necessary factor for career socialisation, advancement and success. Claims have been made that mentors:

- Make good leaders (Zaleznik, 1977; Pelletier & Duffield, 1994)
- Are required for success in business (Collins & Scott, 1978; Segerman-Peck, 1991)
- Are needed for executive success (Roche, 1979; Conway, 1996)
- Lead to scholarliness (May et al., 1982; Sands et al., 1991)

- Are a key to the future of nursing professionalism (Cooper, 1990)
- Can help in tackling social exclusion (Community Care, 1998).

This chapter aims to introduce the mentor and mentoring through an exploration of the differing interpretations for this interesting role and unique relationship in business, education and health care. A conceptual view will be offered in attempts to discover the nature of mentoring via an analysis of the functions, roles and relationships that identify this significant and dynamic, professional support relationship.

What is mentoring?

Mentoring continues to be in vogue and everyone has a mentor or is beginning to want one; however the question remains – is the concept clearly understood? What is a mentor, how do they function, and what are the complexities of the mentoring processes involved? These are questions that need to be addressed if appropriate and viable mentoring systems are to be developed and evaluated. As recently reported, there remains 'considerable semantic and conceptual variability about what mentoring is and does, and what a mentor is and does (SCOPME, 1998, p.5). To separate the myths from the mystique of mentoring is crucial, and we have to consider the origins, influences, approaches, terminology and the variety of different contexts in which mentoring has become visible.

Origins

The term 'mentor' is derived from the Classics, as identified in Homer's *Odyssey* where Mentor, the trusted son of Alimus, was appointed by Ulysses to be tutor–adviser to his son, Telemachus, and guardian of his estates while he was away fighting the Trojan wars. Mentor became more than a guardian, teacher and adviser as he had considerable influence and personal responsibility for the development of the young Telemachus. However, whether Mentor fulfilled his responsibilities diligently and was successful in the role is in doubt, as Homer further informs us that the goddess Athena assumed the disguise of Mentor to act as adviser to the youth. Safire (1980) suggests it was all a trick and that Homer was sending a warning to look out for mentors! It could be, however, that the poet was drawing attention to the complex nature of the relationship, suggesting that there was more to the role than being an older, wiser, adviser of first impressions. There are other scholars who suggest it was all a myth and that Homer's work has been badly misinterpreted in the literature (Playdon, 1998).

It was common in ancient Greece for young males to be partnered with older, experienced males who were often relatives or friends of the family. It was expected that the youths would learn from and emulate the values of their assigned 'mentor'. The term mentor became synonymous with wise, faithful guardian and teacher (Hamilton, 1981).

Roman generals had mentors by their side on the field of battle to advise them, and there are links with mentorship in the master crafts-man–apprenticeship unions of mediaeval times. Guild masters were not only responsible for the teaching of particular crafts but also for their apprentices' social, religious and personal habits.

Few references to mentoring appear in the literature until a resurgence of interest was generated by Levinson's seminal study of adult development (Levinson *et al.*, 1978). The mentor was identified as normally older, of greater experience and more senior in the world that the young man was entering. This mentor was viewed as a transitional, exemplar figure in a young male's development. This was built on in business, education and nursing with the result that mentors and mentoring have been firing the imagination of many occupational groups and professions in recent years (Vance, 1982; Monaghan & Lunt, 1992).

Mentoring terms

The literature is full of various labels for the mentor and mentee (individuals involved) and mentoring or mentorship (the process). The identified labels within a structured, mentoring programme appear to reflect the organisational culture, management style, philosophy or mission of a particular organisation. In health care individuals who are being mentored are described as mentees or students. Murray and Owen (1991) document popular labels in other organisational settings as 'apprentice', 'aspirant', 'advisee', 'counselee', 'trainee', 'protégé' and 'candidate'. Less popular terms are 'follower', 'subordinate', 'applicant', 'hopeful', 'seeker' and we would add 'pupil', 'ward', 'novice', 'novitiate' and 'initiate', which could be considered limiting and judgmental in the mentoring context.

Influences

Moves towards providing organisational support systems that place importance on personal growth and development have roots in a variety of different movements of the 1970s and 1980s. The emergence of management theory and the role of management as a distinct discipline have played a part. However, the major influences appear to have been the human resource development initiatives of the 1970s (Eng, 1986) and the acceptance of freedom-to-learn approaches and adult learning theories of Rogers (1983), Kolb (1984) and Knowles (1984). The resulting shift in organisational and educational philosophies has led to the search for effective strategies that are directed towards making the most of human potential and stimulating learning in practice. The emphasis on being self-directed and *owning* the learning experience has increased responsibility for self learning, self awareness and problem solving, which arises from the acceptance of the theoretical assumptions of adult development and maturation. This involves acknowledging that adults can:

- Move from a state of dependence to become self directed – able to take responsibility for their own actions, self development and life-long learning.
- Accumulate experiences – being able to build a biography of experience that can be drawn on to test and evaluate new experiences. This leads to the search for new learning opportunities, resulting in abilities to learn, change and provide a rich resource for themselves and others.
- Have an orientation towards personal developmental and professional roles, demonstrating a willingness to learn and seek guidance as necessary.
- Change from needing to acquire knowledge and being subject-centred to becoming more performance-centred, resulting in the application of experience and the development of sound critical thinking abilities.

Underpinning these assumptions is the notion that individual growth is perceived as a process of becoming, and not as a process of being shaped or cloned. It is important to realise that self experience and self discovery are important facets of learning (Rogers, 1983.) Adults have built-in motivations to learn, and a need to gain in self-confidence, self-esteem and self-awareness. These are important attributes for any occupational or professional group but are crucial for those caring for the health needs of others. Self-awareness is also an important and necessary prerequisite for 'appreciating self and the situation of others' (Burnard, 1988, p. 229). This is a vital component of personal growth and development and it fits well with the 'process of becoming' as a continual journey of self discovery. Assistance, offered by a confident, self-secure, experienced guide and enabler in the form of a mentor, can aid the keen, inexperienced traveller.

The *raison d'être* of mentoring

Mentoring is an exciting complex phenomenon that is natural or artificially contrived to benefit individuals within a sharing partnership (Palmer, 1987). In the true classical sense it is much more than the experienced guiding the inexperienced: mentoring is dynamic and exciting, in part because of its kaleidoscopic nature and also because it is a relatively complex concept, made more intricate by the various connotations placed on it. It is a good example of a transcendental semantic signifier – taken in this context to mean that mentoring can be viewed from many different perspectives and is open to a variety of interpretations depending on its differing applications and settings.

Mentoring concerns the building of a dynamic relationship in which the personal characteristics, philosophies and priorities of the individual members interact to influence, in turn, the nature, direction and duration of the resulting, eventual partnership. What lies at the heart of the process is the shared, encouraging and supportive elements that are based on mutual attraction and common values. It is these aspects that facilitate the personal development and career/professional socialisation for the mentee – leading to eventual reciprocal benefits for both parties.

A mentoring relationship is one that is enabling and cultivating, a relationship that assists in empowering an individual within the working environment. A mentor is not a prerequisite for advancement or success as such events regularly occur without access to this type of significant helper. It is important to recognise that mentors do not have magic abilities or powers to fashion great individuals (Fields, 1991). They do, however, enable individuals to discover and use their own talents, encouraging and nurturing the unique contributions of their mentees, to help them be successful in their own right.

Mentoring is concerned with making the most of human potential and significantly is becoming more widely recognised in health care at a time of political change and with moves away from competitive, market approaches towards collaborative practices (DoH, 1997). As part of an identified support framework of other more recognisable roles and staff development programmes, mentoring fits well with humanistic management, education and training initiatives. This involves adult approaches and learning experiences supported by the principles of self-development, self-directedness, mutual understanding and negotiation.

However, in the British health service and the general and higher education systems, currently concerned with diminishing resources, efficiency and value for money, mentoring mechanisms of a more formalised nature may rest more easily within the prevailing ethos. For the clinical manager, educator, lecturer, staff developer or researcher, mentoring presents an intriguing challenge when considering the what, how and where of practical application.

Mentoring challenges

On examining mentoring it rapidly becomes apparent that the views from a variety of perspectives, and the lack of clarity of purposes and functions of the mentor, are not assisted by anecdotal reports, lack of empirical evidence and confusion with other professional support roles. What remains crucial in today's climate is a need to come to terms with the nature of new support roles and then to apply them appropriately. This is important with regard to the types of approaches that are available and may be required.

Important questions to be considered include who needs, wants or will benefit from such new roles? Making informed decisions about what systems are required and how they should be planned, implemented, evaluated and resourced will enable managers, educators and those from staff development units to make adequate preparations to assist staff to come to terms with new support roles, structures and frameworks.

It would be easy to step into the 'quagmire of definitions' envisaged by Hagerty (1986). It is far better to clarify the roles that already exist and to consider the nature of the classical mentor as interpreted by Levinson *et al.* (1978). This leads to the discovery of the richness of the relationship and facilitates an explanation of the various mentoring approaches that exist. Informed decisions and choices can then be made regarding the development of sound mentoring frameworks to complement the other organisational support systems that are available.

The classical mentor

In reviewing mentoring it soon becomes apparent that common elements underpin the different perspectives, cultures and approaches. Vance (1982) helps to clarify the situation by drawing attention to the earlier suggestions arising from business studies, that mentoring is not defined in the identification of formal roles but in the character of the relationship and the function it serves. Business, education and nursing applications of mentoring may initially appear different in terminology, focus and approachs; however, certain common elements emerge. These can be identified as:

- The character of the relationship is that of enabling and empowerment
- The mentor offers a repertoire of helper functions (or assisting functions) to facilitate guidance and provide support
- The mentor role comprises an interplay of personal, functional and relational aspects
- Individual purposes and helper functions are mutually set by the individuals involved
- Helper functions are mutually determined by the individuals
- Individuals choose each other and there are identifiable stages in the relationship.

Character of the relationship

In classical mentoring the central focus of the partnership concerns the mutual trust of two adult individuals attracted by the possibility of what has been described as a mentor signal (George & Kummerow, 1981). The two parties are drawn together naturally by their personal characteristics, attributes and common values. They demonstrate a willingness to spend time together, to learn from each other and to share each other's experiences.

In the early stages of the relationship the mentee may appear initially dependent or reliant on the mentor in terms of the intensity of the support offered. As the relationship develops there will be changes in the intensity as the needs and priorities of the mentee change. This results in an intimacy to the relationship made possible by mutual relevance and closeness and a reciprocal partnership develops into one that is dynamic, emotionally intense and beneficial to each party.

Recognition of the partnership, and better understanding of his/her own needs, allows the mentee to become proactive in triggering the specific support or assistance required. The mentee can begin to be self-selecting with regard to the helper functions required and can begin to make informed decisions about personal development.

Testing, taking risks, making mistakes and the freedom to be creative take place within the mutual understanding that the mentee is valued and supported. Safety mechanisms exist in the form of the wide range of helper functions offered the mentor. The mentee becomes gradually more self-aware, gains in confidence and begins to achieve the capacity to 'go it alone'. It is at this stage that he/she may look for another mentor or become a mentor to someone else.

In this manner the classical mentor facilitates personal growth and development and assists with career progression, while guiding the mentee through the clinical, educational, social and political networks of the working culture. The elements of mentoring that set it apart from other more specific relationships and give it its multidimensional and dynamic nature are the:

- Repertoire of helper functions
- Mutuality and reciprocal sharing
- Duration, identified stages and transitional nature of the relationship.

These required elements match with Darling's (1984) vital ingredients for mentoring, which she identifies as attraction, action and effect.

Repertoire of helper functions

Within work, individuals may develop relationships that are specific in nature such as role modelling, teaching or counselling. These relationships are clearly defined and are considered functionally specific. If a deeper association develops with mutual attraction, and the wide range of helper functions is offered, then the relationship becomes dynamic, reciprocal and emotionally intense, and true, classical mentoring occurs (Palmer, 1987, p. 36.) The emotional aspect arises from an intimacy that is made possible by the closeness and understanding of those involved. The helper functions of mentoring are:

- Adviser
- Coach
- Counsellor
- Guide/networker
- Role model
- Sponsor
- Teacher
- Resource facilitator

Adviser

Support and advice is offered in both career and social terms. The advice given demonstrates an awareness of the mentee's merits and abilities within the organisation's requirements. This process aids in building the self-image and confidence of the mentee.

Coach

In mentoring, the coaching function concerns the mutual setting of guidelines with the mentor offering advice and constructive feedback.

The mentee can then test such feedback in differing practice situations. The mutual exchange between the individuals allows feedback to be analysed and refined for future action.

Counsellor

The role of counsellor facilitates self-development of the mentee in his/ her own terms as psychological support systems are made available. The mentor acts as a listener and sounding-board to facilitate self-awareness and encourage independence.

Guide/networker

As a supportive guide, the mentor introduces the mentee to the helpful contacts and power groups within the organisation. Networking is an extension of guiding as the mentor facilitates introductions to the values and customs of the organisation, including socialisation to the mentor's own occupational, professional and social groups.

Role model

A role model provides an observable image for imitation, demonstrating skills and qualities for the mentee to emulate.

Sponsor

The sponsor influences and facilitates entry to the organisational and professional cultures. The mentor influences career development by providing introductions, promoting the mentee and making recommendations for advancement.

Teacher

The teacher function involves sharing knowledge through experience and critical inquiry, facilitating learning opportunities, and focusing on individual needs and learning styles to promote ownership and responsibility for continuing professional education. Such activities and reflection on experience assist personal development, in order to fulfil intellectual and practical potential.

Resource facilitator

The mentor acts as an experienced practitioner and colleague sharing experiences and information, as well as providing access to resources.

This forms the preceptor-type, resource element within the range of helper functions.

Personal, functional and relational factors

The personal and relational factors are concerned with individual growth, self-development, self-awareness and personal fulfilment. Knowing that there is someone out there willing to offer support and encouragement and 'in their corner' enables the mentee to come to terms with his/her role in the organisation or professional setting. The mentor offers personal, functional and relational assistance to provide a comprehensive framework of support that goes beyond those of the more usual teaching and advisory roles in clinical practice. Within such a framework the mentee can begin to constructively question his/her own abilities and can gain in confidence, be creative and endeavour to take risks. The inter-relationship of these personal, functional and relational factors is identified in Table 2.1.

Table 2.1 The support framework of personal, functional and relational factors within mentoring.

| | Mentor Role | |
Personal	Functional	Relational
promoting	*providing*	*facilitating*
self development	teaching	interpersonal relations
confidence building	coaching	social relations
creativity	role modelling	networking
fulfilment of potential	counselling	sharing
risk taking	support	trust
	advice	
	sponsorship	
	guidance	
	resources	

Mutual setting of individual purposes and functions

Jointly attracted by each other's qualities and attributes, in classical mentoring the mentor and mentee are free to develop the relationship in the manner of their choosing. The emphasis is on informality, and the needs of the individuals concerned form the character and nature of the resulting relationship. The mentee can feel safe in selecting particular helper functions that are required in his/her own terms, while moving from initial dependency in the relationship to becoming independent and his/her own person.

In classical mentoring informal assessment may exist in the tentative, early phases of the partnership but only in the form of evaluating each other's experiences, abilities, approachability and willingness to find time for each other. It is our considered opinion that formal assessment and documentation procedures have no place in this type of mentoring.

Mentor language, functions and organisational culture

In classical mentoring, it is important to recognise that the nature and terms of the relationship are set informally by the people involved. The nature of the relationship is determined by the qualities and characteristics of the people drawn together through the sharing of common values or attitudes to form an initial attraction and bonding. The processes which evolve are formulated by both parties, naturally occurring and informal within the specific organisational culture. The expectations and any issues that arise will relate to what the mentor and mentee may deem as important in gaining the 'tribal wisdom' of an organisation, (Darling, 1984) or obtaining the 'DNA of a profession' (Palmer, 1992).

The expectations include the need for active participation and developmental outcomes tailored to the needs of the mentee to provide a sharing, collaborative partnership that benefits both individuals and the organisation or relevant occupational group or profession.

The nature of the relationship will be affected by the organisational culture that consists of the values, norms and beliefs of the structures and systems that give an organisation its own identity (Handy, 1985; Cray & Mallory, 1998). In classical mentoring the relationship is inherently of their own making and not artificially contrived. Modifications to classical mentoring in order to fulfil a variety of differing individual and organisational requirements have led to the application of more formal approaches. The true elements of classical mentoring (mutuality, repertoire of helper functions, duration) may well be evident but there will be adaptations and a differing emphasis placed on career support, socialisation and the criteria for success.

In more formal forms of mentoring such as contract (Monaghan & Lunt, 1992) or facilitated mentoring (Murray & Owen, 1991), mentor terminology and helper functions are determined by the organisational culture (refer to Table 2.2 for an explanation of approaches). Contract mentoring concerns the adaptation of classical mentoring and its resulting application within structured programmes of support. The people involved are obliged to achieve the identified aims, purposes and outcomes of a recognised programme of development and support. The

Table 2.2   Mentoring approaches.

Type	Nature
1. True mentoring relationships	
(i) Classical mentoring – informal. (Primary mentoring) A natural, chosen relationship. Purposes and functions are determined by the individuals involved. An enabling relationship in personal, emotional, organisational and professional terms.	• Self-selection of individuals, persuasive influences; attraction with a shared wish to work together. • No defined programme. • Less specific purposes and functions as set by the individuals, circumstances and context. • No explicit financial rewards for mentor. • Probable duration, 2–15 years.
(ii) Contract mentoring – formal. (Facilitated mentoring/secondary mentoring) An artificial relationship created for a specific purpose, that is essentially determined by the organisation. Some elements of mentor function, with focus on specific helper functions.	Programmes are identified by: • Clear purposes, functions, defined aims or outcomes. • Selected individuals with assigned mentors, forced matiching or choice of mentors from mentor pool. • Explicit material rewards; possibilities of financial incentives for mentors. • Probable duration, 1–2 years.
2. Pseudo-mentoring relationships (Quasi mentoring/partial mentoring/ sequential mentoring) Mentoring approaches in appearance only – as offered by academic involvement in thesis preparation, orientation and induction programmes.	• Focus on specific tasks or organisational issues of short lived duration. • Guidance from several mentors, for short periods. • Relationships do not demonstrate the comprehensive enabling elements of the true classical model. • Specified clinical placements. • Probable duration, 6 weeks to one year.

relevant aims, purposes and outcomes may or may not be negotiable, depending on the degree of formality of the programme. Individuals can be assigned to each other (forced matching) or may be able to make a choice from a selected group of mentors, known as the 'mentor pool'. These issues will be explored later in the chapter.

The nature of the process may have superficial similarities within different organisations or within differing occupational groups, but how the process is explained and understood may take on a variety of appearances. Often formulated for organisational requirements as part of staff development programmes, the use of different terminology and the change in emphasis for the helper functions give rise to the different approaches of mentoring that are evident within differing cultures.

Classical mentoring and contract mentoring can be considered as true mentoring as both contain the vital elements essential to mentoring: the helper functions, mutuality and sharing and identified stages/duration. Pseudo-mentoring or quasi-mentoring approaches have probably arisen due to the initial lack of understanding of the roles, purposes, processes and formal application of mentoring.

Early applications tended to confuse mentoring with the support provided by preceptors, academic counsellors and personal tutors. Mentoring was also used for the singular purposes of orientation and induction, where the richness of the relationship is wasted and more functional enabling roles such as preceptorship would suffice. (An elaboration of pseudo-mentoring is given in Table 2.2.)

Organisational applications in business and education

In business, the emphasis is for the mentor to function as a sponsor, guide or networker within a competitive culture that is often male dominated (Demarco, 1993). The main focus has been on career guidance, executive nurturing and managerial support, with informal or formal, planned programmes of contract/facilitated mentoring (Murray & Owen, 1991). Mentoring in business organisations is considered to have a place in developing potential managers and executives, as well as having a strategic role in managing change and implementing new work practices (Slipais, 1993; Conway, 1996).

In the USA, business interest in mentoring systems stimulated education policy makers and educators to consider such approaches for student preparation, teachers and school administrators (Klopf & Harrison, 1981; Fagan & Walter, 1982.) The focus for mentor function was essentially that of teacher and role model with educational aims that were adapted from those of business to reduce the accent on financial rewards. Education has become more concerned with the process of learning, resulting in roles for educators that stimulate adult learning and reflection, altering the balance of power towards the learning needs of the student.

In general education in the UK, the focus for mentoring programmes was initially conceived for educational and pastoral support in probationary periods. Scant further interest was taken in the concept, despite the recommendations of the James Committee (James Report, 1972). Later in the 1970s the Advisory Committee on the Supply and Training of Teachers (ACSTT) set up a subcommittee, chaired by Professor Haycocks, which subsequently produced three influential reports. The second subcommittee report on the training of adult education and part-time further education teachers (ACSTT II), which became more popularly known as Haycocks II, reported in March 1978.

One of the report's recommendations centred on the provision of a local team of mentors to play a part in offering a role as classroom counsellors in teacher training. Holt (1982, p. 153), in valuing such a proposal for 'on-course, in-house support', identified difficulties in implementation because of cost, mentor training and the effectiveness of the supervisory role in the classroom.

Beyond initial school education, the envisaged changes had implications for general staff development, providing 'training for the trainers' and for those involved in further education (Cantor & Roberts, 1986, p.192). Current interest has once again arisen due to the changes in initial teacher training programmes and the increase in school-based training as part of initial teacher training (Department for Education, 1992; Boydell & Bines, 1994; Tomlinson, 1995). Student teachers are located in educational placements and are expected to learn 'on the job', with support from a qualified teacher acting as a mentor.

In primary education, mentoring for student teachers has tended to take the form of collaborative relationship's which facilitate openness, the sharing of feelings and professional issues (Boydell, 1994). Mentoring has continued to gain momentum in secondary education with the introduction of school-based initial teacher training/education schemes. As a result an interesting discourse has been and is taking place, with the sharing of widely differing interpretations and applications for the mentor in general and higher education (Standing, 1999).

Glover *et al.* (1994) with evidence from a wide scale study on mentoring have uncovered what they consider are the three determinants that affect the mentoring process. These are identified as the subject mentor, the subject department and the staff of the school, and it is suggested that the balance of these three factors has the greatest effect on the mentoring relationship and student experience. A rational and useful explanation for the development and current explosion of mentor interpretations in education is offered by Brooks & Sikes (1997), who trace the application of the various emerging models which complement the 'classical' approach. Such models are identifiable as the three types offered here.

(1) The apprenticeship model and the mentor as skilled crafts person

Practical applications:

- Pupil–apprentice and teacher–master roles
- Learning by observing, 'sitting by Nellie'
- For initial teacher training mode (O'Hear, 1988).

There have been some adaptions to this model and there is recognition for the change in language from apprenticeship to that of 'modelling' (McIntyre, 1994). This it would appear provides a useful and supportive relationship when identified circumstances dictate the need for security at the start of a course.

(2) The competence-based model and the mentor as trainer

Practical applications:

- Training and induction with the role of the trainer as an instructor and coach who demonstrates and assists the student to achieve a set of competencies, as identified by the Department for Education (1992, para 2.1). Parsloe (1995) explains the coaching role well and makes helpful links with the development of competencies.

(3) The reflective practitioner model and mentor as critical friend and co-enquirer

Practical applications:

- Promoting collaboration and partnership in the learning process
- The notion of challenge to promote professional growth.

This mode of mentoring in general secondary education initiates learning from experience, with reflection, 'in and on action', to assist new teachers with the complexities of their teaching role and the 'swampy lowlands of professional practice (Schon, 1988). This type of mentoring relationship fits well with the notion of quality mentoring forwarded by Fish (1995) who makes links with the need for reflective practice as well as a healthy balance of the process and skills required to be a competent and 'quality mentor'.

Application to health care

In British health care, supportive role developments have been many and varied with occupational groups such as social workers and occupational therapists devising structured, sound, clinical enabling relationships that develop therapeutic competence (Hawkins & Shohet, 1989, CCETSW, 1992). Such relationships and supervisory support roles assist training and facilitate assessment in practical placements, as well as support advanced practice. Modifications of therapeutically determined supervisory roles allow learning support to be provided by practising field work teachers, supervisors and community trainers. Those in physio-therapy and the complementary therapies such as acupuncture also recognise a need for students to experience professional work, enabling them to re-examine practice effectively through investigation, analysis and professional support (Pratt, 1989; MacPherson, 1997).

Supervision appears to be the identified learning support role for the therapies and social work disciplines, particularly for those on training programmes, while mentors have responsibility for supporting the qualified worker (Rumsey, 1995). In radiography and medicine, men-toring is steadily being explored (Barr *et al.*, 1993; Bould, 1996) and further information on how these and other health occupations provide learning support and supervisory frameworks will be discussed in Chapter 4.

Despite comprehensive activity in north America, in the UK only a few mentor programmes for senior managers have been instigated (Muller, 1984; Holloran, 1993). For the most part in the National Health Service at present, mentoring is 'provided' for student nurses and student midwives and 'faculty mentors' were recommended for medical students (Calkins, *et al.*, 1987). In British nursing and midwifery, mentoring issues have been further complicated by the confusion over the role and functions of other support roles – preceptor and clinical supervisors.

It is well documented that the terms mentor and preceptor were brought to the consciousness of most British nurses via the educational language and curriculum developments of the 1990s. The nursing origi-nators who set the scene for the take up of the concept in the UK were mainly North American authors, consultants and researchers, notably Vance (1982), Darling (1984) and Puetz (1985). Most admit to having drawn on the experiences of the business and commercial arenas where the empirical evidence has involved mostly male experiences in the world of work and has concentrated on leadership development.

Nursing, midwifery and the other health care professions remain primarily female and transferring empirical and anecdotal evidence from different cultures can further complicate understanding and application. There are fundamental differences of product–process ethos between business and service organisations like the health service which has imperatives for setting social objectives and 'managing for social result' (Weil, 1992; Morley, 1995). In nursing, important mentoring issues of cross gender approaches and some female nurses' lack of apparent abilities to network, share and support emerging leaders have been readily addressed (Hamilton 1981; Hardy 1984). There is evidence that nurses are gaining in assertiveness and increased political acumen in other countries but in Britain gender remains a key factor in how nurses value their health care contribution (Davies, 1995).

The word 'mentor' first appeared in the curriculum preparation documents produced by one of the statutory bodies, the English National Board (ENB, 1987, 1988). New roles were rapidly created and new name badges worn with some pride and a great deal of puzzlement for both qualified staff and students alike. The use of the term preceptor, again with its origins in North America, had appeared earlier in the nursing index for 1975 and in popular nursing press reports, where a scheme was developed within one health authority (Raichura & Riley, 1985).

The use of preceptors has once again been brought to notice by the stated intentions of the Post-Registration Education and Practice initiatives (PREP), which explore the requirements for continual updating, post-registration support and the development of appropriate portfolios of practice achievements (UKCC, 1995). Critical examination by British authors and researchers has continually highlighted the need to use preceptors appropriately in the clinical setting (Morle, 1990; Barlow, 1991) and it has been noticeable that nursing authors switched emphasis from discussing the merits of mentorship to comparing and contrasting both roles and how they could best be used (Armitage & Burnard, 1991; Ashton & Richardson, 1992).

Clarity about the nature of the different roles has not been helped by early articles that attempted to describe mentoring but with the benefit of hindsight were describing preceptorship programmes or pseudo-mentoring approaches. Morle (1990) concluded that current role definition is probably inappropriate and nursing would be better advised to use the term 'preceptor', a role more oriented and suited to practice. What is important in the current debate in nursing is that mentoring, preceptorship and the emerging professional support role of clinical supervision, should all be seen to have equal value for development and support in whichever setting they are applied.

Mentoring in medicine is steadily gaining credence and, after a late start in comparison with the other health care groups, has begun to identify suitable guidance for the role of mentoring within continuing medical education. Recognition has been forthcoming for a number of years concerning the need for support in all branches of medicine and the importance for effective continuing education (SCOPME, 1997; Freeman, 1998).

However, it is only relatively recently that mentoring has been viewed as a pivotal relationship in supporting the various grades of doctor. Mentoring in general practice schemes has highlighted the tensions and dilemmas between providing pastoral support or educational support (Alliott, 1996) and a range of mentoring activities have been identified including that of the 'holistic' mentor (Freeman, 1997). The holistic mentor is thought to bind together the classical components of mentoring which the author and researcher considers are continuing professional education, personal support and professional development (Freeman, 1997, p. 457).

A new study offers clarity of definition and sound conclusions are reached to assist the implementation of mentoring in medicine and dentistry. Mentoring, it is suggested, involves 'a process whereby an experienced, highly regarded, empathetic person (the mentor) guides another individual in the development and re-examination of their own ideas, learning and personal and professional development' (SCOPME, 1998, p. 12). If mentoring is to become a successful, worthwhile activity the authors of the report conclude that there is a need for:

- Dissemination of mentoring's potential benefits, risks, aims and processes
- Promotion of opportunities for mentoring, but it should not be imposed
- Identification of mentoring as a priority for newly appointed career grade doctors and dentists
- Development and evaluation of preparation programmes for those volunteering to become mentors
- Clarity of initiatives developed locally and nationally
- View of mentoring as a positive, enabling experience separate and distinct from organisational systems of monitoring or performance review.

Mentoring is coming of age in the medical profession, having learnt from the early confusions and pseudo-mentoring approaches still being agonised over in nursing. However, small pockets of mentoring initiatives will have to be nurtured and traditional cultures of 'difficult rites of passage' will have to be addressed, if the full potential of this enabling relationship is to be realised in both secondary and primary health care.

Choice and mentoring stages

Individual selection is a vital process of classical mentoring as the relationship is dependent on the joint, dynamic, sharing characteristics of both parties for its nature and success. Matching characteristics and a 'coming together' are naturally implied in the mentor signal and common attraction that ignites the relationship. Enjoyment of each other's company and a willingness to spend time together may signal the start to this informal mentoring process. Styles of approach and the individual preferences of both parties play their part in how the 'personal fit' is best made (Klopf & Harrison, 1981).

Phases or stages to the relationship are variously described and documented and these are commonly identified as the initiation, development and termination phases (Campbell-Heider, 1986; Earnshaw, 1995). Others suggest that there are four phases and clarify these as: initiation, training and termination with the establishment of lasting peer friendship as a follow-up to an amicable ending (Hunt & Michael, 1983).

In nursing, Hawkins & Thibodeau (1989) specify invitational, questioning, informational/working and termination stages. Common to many of the deliberations on the phases or stages is the fact that the relationship is transitional and there is always a recognisable start, middle and end to any mentoring relationship.

Initiation

The start or initiation concerns the 'locking on' of individuals who are brought together by common characteristics, abilities or recognition of shared values. This involves the selection and 'getting to know you' period of the relationship. Working in close proximity, having access to each other and being able to observe each other's actions in a variety of work situations, influences the initial attraction and assists the 'coming together' phase.

Working phase

The working or training phase of the process is where the main focus for individual growth and development lies. The dynamics of the mentoring relationship are maintained by the interactions of both individuals and the increasing trust and closeness that begins to develop. The mentee may commence this phase by being heavily reliant on the mentor's greater experience, awareness of the networks and wide variety of influential contacts.

The mentee is faced with the repertoire of helper functions that the experienced mentor has to offer and the choice of assistance may initially be erratic and left to chance. As this phase develops, mutual trust and sharing become evident and the mentee is more readily able to choose the specific helper functions that are best suited to his/her needs. This is a very active phase and the intensity of the relationship moves to that of common understanding and solid partnership. The mentee gradually becomes more independent and is eventually able to trigger or request the specific helper functions required.

Through the mutual sharing of experiences and needs, the mentee is able to make informed decisions and become self-selecting within the relationship. Figure 2.1 shows the mentoring phases with relevant activities and degree of attachment. The transitional nature of the relationship sets the scene for the mentee to have the confidence to be creative and to experiment with risk-taking ventures that further encourage growth and development.

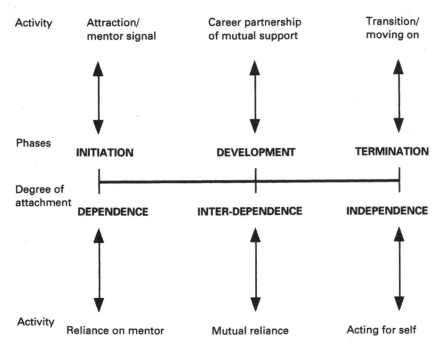

Fig. 2.1 Matching phases of mentoring with activities and degree of attachment.

The need to test and take risks arises within the understanding that the mentee is valued and supported and that there are safety measures available should mistakes occur. The mentee becomes increasingly more confident to go it alone and the relationship moves towards the terminating phase.

Termination phase

The mentee has begun to act on his/her own initiative and is now in a position to begin to act independently. The termination phase can end positively as supportive friendship or negatively where there is conflict or emotional tension and general dissatisfaction (Blotnick, 1984; Wheatley & Hirsch, 1984). The ending can be precipitated by changing career interests, a need to find another mentor or to take on the challenges of mentoring others, or the emergence of toxic mentoring. (This is explored more fully in the benefits and limitations of mentoring dealt with later in this chapter.)

If the process has been beneficial with the identified needs being met, the two individuals may maintain their friendship and the mentee may move on to mentor others. This may be due in part to the need for another association that involves sharing or a desire for a degree of emotional intensity that is not always readily available within other working relationships.

Attributes, qualities and abilities of an effective mentor

Just as there is no single definition for a mentor, there is no single personality type that is synonymous with being or becoming an effective mentor. But it is evident that successful mentors are reported as employing a range of enabling strategies and skills within mentoring relationships (Fields, 1991; Anderson & Shannon, 1995). In considering who should mentor it is important to consider the behaviours, qualities and characteristics of those who will be deemed suitable to provide this supportive role for others. The intention is not to be prescriptive but to present some idea of what is meant by positive strategies in order to assist managers, educators and practitioners in making a sound selection. This will aid the deliberations about who is best fitted to support others and who requires help in attaining appropriate qualities, and it will perhaps identify those who should never be placed in a position to support or mentor others.

In this chapter and those that follow, a common theme in the discussion is the use of the term 'enabling', – epitomising the positive aspects of human relationships that foster growth and development in others. 'Enabling' refers to the ability to make things happen and in recent years it has become associated with the other positive development concepts of facilitation and empowerment. The working world would be vastly different if organisations were staffed and managed solely by people with these enabling qualities. The richness, complexity and challenges of the working culture are, however, diversified by the fact that human beings are capable of displaying both enabling and disabling qualities.

Disabling traits

In examining of the nature of support roles it is necessary to reflect on the less positive aspects of human nature that can have a detrimental effect on others. Having identified individuals in management systems who are disruptive, Heirs and Farrell (1986) categorise these individuals who through their thought processes and actions typify aspects of disabling behaviour. The 'destructive minds' are categorised by the following features:

The rigid mind:
- Concrete thinkers, dealing with only black and white concepts
- Stereotyped, with preconceived ideas that are difficult to change
- Set values, which lack imagination or creativity
- In authority, stifle others, suspicious and resistant to new ideas
- Safe and secure in bureaucratic surroundings.

The rigid mind: stifles originality, ignores change and encourages complacency.

The ego mind:
- Self interested and self important
- Uninterested in others and keen to always get their own way
- Unable to share
- Destroys team cohesiveness and spirit
- Works well as an outsider or entrepreneur.

The ego mind: destroys objectivity and makes 'thinking collaboration' impossible.

The machiavellian mind:
- Devious, calculating and manipulative
- Obsessed by internal politics and politicking' Heirs & Farrell, 1986, p.182)
- Interested in power and power plays.

The machiavellian mind turns all thinkers into bureaucratic connivers and all thinking into political thinking.

Heirs and Farrell suggest that we should learn to manage these individuals and attempt to understand how they operate. However, if this is not possible then Heirs and Farrell advise avoiding them, taking care that they do not 'infect' your thinking (Heirs & Farrell, 1986, p.86).

Vera Darling (1986), in taking a slightly different perspective, offers a 'galaxy of toxic mentors', developed from interviewing nurses. Four distinct types of disabler are observed and these she refers to as the avoiders, dumpers, blockers and destroyer/criticisers. This informal classification and the associated subgroups are presented in overview in Table 2.3. The apparent behaviours have similarities to those presented by the 'destructive minds' and these are clearly not the qualities expected of an enabler or those we would wish to identify as effective in supporting others. They present as those clearly at the other end of a continuum of positive supporting strategies.

Table 2.3 The galaxy of toxic mentors.

Type	Features
Dumpers	Not available or accessible Throw people into new roles Leave them to 'sink or swim' strategies

Blockers	Avoid meeting others' needs by:
	  refusing requests ('the Refuser')
	  controlling through withholding information ('the Withholder')
	  arresting development by over supervising ('the Hoverer')

Destroyer/Criticisers	Set out to destroy others by:
	  subtle attacks to undermine confidence ('the Underminer')
	  open approaches of verbal attack and argument to deliberately destroy confidence ('the Belittler') constant put-downs and questioning of abilities ('the Nagger')

Source: Darling (1985).

Rather than present a continuum of positive support with polarisations of enabling and disabling traits, which gives the appearance of being relatively simple and of one dimension, another positive attribute, facilitation, can be added to the equation, along with that of another negative trait, such as manipulation. The resulting perspectives demonstrate the rich diversities of enabling and disabling characteristics that can occur. This is demonstrated in Fig. 2.2, where the positive qualities of enabling are in opposition to those of the negative disabling. These in turn are counter-balanced by the positive nature of facilitation and the negativity of manipulation.

This completes the four quadrants, and the entities of the enablers, disablers and those that fall between – the enabling manipulator (enabling-disabler) and disabling facilitator (disabling-enabler) – emerge. Although it is relatively easy to spot the true enablers and disablers within an organisation, it is not always so easy to identify the negative and detrimental effects of those who are enabling-disablers or disabling-

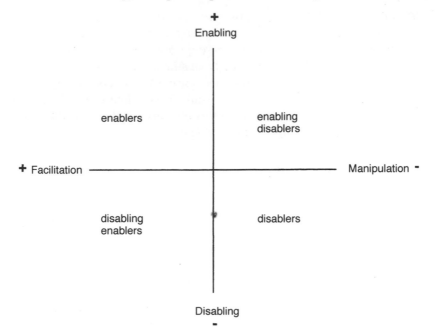

Fig. 2.2   Enabling–disabling traits.

enablers. Often these individuals present with a much more subtle approach, and it may take some time to realise that a relationship that appears as initially sound is, in fact, disabling and having a negative effect.

The disablers fit with Darling's description of dumpers and blockers while the enabling-disablers and disabling-enablers are easily recognisable within the category of destroyers and criticisers. By creating tensions and disruptions they can cause others to move departments or change jobs; conversely, enablers may create too comfortable an existence that is reassuring and seducing. That is not to say that these behaviours are tolerated, rather that an understanding of how they operate can help us work with, manage and draw those who demonstrate disabling traits towards the beneficial effects of a supportive relationship.

Enabling traits

Having dealt with the negative aspects we can now focus on the more positive elements. An enabler is someone who appears as an open, honest communicator, a person who feels positive about him/herself and about his/her value to the organisation and to others within it. Enablers are people-centred and because they feel worthy and can value themselves, they are in turn able to recognise the value of others. An enabling individual is:

- Accessible to those around him/her
- Responsive to others' needs
- Easy to trust
- Comfortable with him/herself and his/her abilities
- Able to command mutual respect.

Other authors list a comprehensive range of characteristics or qualities that appear to be best suited to mentoring as a long-term, close working relationship. Holloway & Whyte (1994, p. 16) identify a checklist for the ideal mentor which includes the attributes of 'relevant job related experience; well developed interpersonal skills; an ability to relate; a desire to assist; an open mind; a flexible attitude and a recognition of their own need for support'.

Extensive lists and tables of the essential ingredients needed to function as an effective mentor can be drawn together within a framework of three important personal attributes. We suggest that these are competence, demonstrating personal confidence, and having a commitment to the development of others. In possessing these personal attributes the mentor has the qualities and abilities to extend a working relationship beyond that of ordinary limits to ensure that mentoring occurs and is effective for all concerned.

Competence

The mentor has competence:

- Arising from having appropriate knowledge and experience to be effective in their work within the organisation and able to command respect from others
- To build on the mentee's strengths and offer constructive feedback on his/her limitations
- In the skills associated with the repertoire of helper functions, such as interpersonal relations, communication, counselling, instructing and coaching, skills that are more value if exercised and up to date
- In providing a reliable source of information and availability of resources
- To promote good judgement.

Confidence

The mentor has confidence to:

- Have and share a network of valuable personal contacts
- Be imaginative
- Demonstrate initiative, take risks and have personal power with charisma that is used appropriately
- Allow the mentee to develop within his/her own terms
- Seek new challenges and initiatives.
- Be successful at what he/she does, providing status and prestige
- Lead and offer clear direction
- Recognise and share credit for achievements
- Be able to deal with another's personal problems, challenges and triumphs.

Commitment

The mentor is committed to:

- Staff development
- Being people orientated and having a keen interest in seeing others develop and advance
- Investing time, energy and effort within a different type of working relationship
- Sharing personal experiences, knowledge and skills
- Personal motivation and a desire to motivate others.

Competence, confidence and commitment ensure that the mentor can be flexible, proactive and responsive, to balance the requisites of a long-term, intimate working relationship with an understanding of its transitional nature and eventual conclusion.

It is also important that the mentor is self-aware with a clear sense of his/her own strengths and limitations, enabling assistance in another's personal growth and development. Positive qualities of flexibility, approachability, accessibility, political astuteness, patience, perseverance and a sense of humour are also essential for effective mentorship. These are sound qualities that ensure that mentors are relatively at ease with themselves, do not take themselves too seriously and can with competence, confidence and commitment be generous towards others, playing their part as an effective enabler and leader. By recognising the differing qualities, needs and aspirations of those around us, we can begin to assist them to value their strengths in becoming part of the team and providing support to others. In summary (modified from the first edition of this book), a mentor has the following characteristics:

Core enabling characteristics – a mentor:
- Motivates individuals to set their own agenda for working and learning
- Provides safe opportunities for critical reflection
- Advises, counsels and guides on personal, professional and career matters
- Assists the mentee to learn through their successes and failures
- Is an effective role model
- Recognises and supports the mentee's strengths
- Develops capabilities by offering constructive feedback.

Specific enabling characteristics – a mentor:
- Is supportive and encouraging
- Helps identify resources for learning and career socialisation
- Is challenging and acts as a critical friend
- Encourages creativity and risk taking in learning and working
- Assists the mentee to critically reflect on his/her personal and professional capabilities.

Qualities for attracting a mentor

Mentoring always concerns two interested parties, with the abilities to form and sustain a working relationship. Although the qualities and skills that a mentor possesses are vital to the nature and effectiveness of the ensuing relationship, the qualities of a mentee also come into play when considering the unfolding of the resulting relationship. The essential ingredients and basic roles to be undertaken are also influenced by the qualities, skills and characteristics of the mentee. Indeed there are those who suggest that there are identifiable strategies that can be employed in attracting a mentor (Zey, 1984, p. 175; Holloway & Whyte, 1994). Qualities that endeavour to make a mentee potentially 'attractive' to a mentor include:

Standing out of the crowd:
- Achieving high visibility
- Having a positive attitude to work or career
- Willing to take risks
- Commitment to own development.

Demonstrating the potential to succeed:
- Willingness to learn and assist the mentor to achieve goals

- Having initiative and motivation
- Ambitious and conscientious
- Receptive to coaching, advice and support.

Adult intimacy capabilities:
- Having a positive self esteem
- Able to make a personal contribution
- Loyal to individuals and the organisation
- Enlightened and enthusiastic
- Making oneself accessible
- Able to make a personal contribution
- Willingness to develop a relationship with the mentor.

Benefits and limitations of mentoring

The benefits

Evidence in the literature suggests that the positive effects are mutually split to benefit the mentor, mentee and organisation (Zey, 1984; Cooper, 1990; Freeman 1997). The strengths and benefits of mentoring arise from the attraction, sharing and developing properties of the relationship. The beneficial effects can be related to degrees of satisfaction for those involved:

- *The mentor:* personal satisfaction and professional development from aiding and abetting another's development
- *The mentee:* professional identity and increased job satisfaction with the possibilities of advancement and success as they become socialised to the organisation
- *The organisation:* a satisfied and motivated workforce with positive outcomes for customers and clients.

Other benefits concern leadership development as the qualities and abilities associated with effective mentoring are synonymous with good leadership. Mentoring can assist in developing leaders, with mentees looked on as emerging leaders, cultivated for their flexibility, adaptability, sound judgment and creativity within an organisation. If mentoring is appropriately recognised as part of the organisational culture, working relationships are very likely to be more open and effective. Such openness improves communication and encourages a greater degree of collegiality and general sharing approaches.

Finally, thoughts should be directed towards the possible constraining factors that may inhibit mentoring from occurring, even if formal pro-grammes of contract mentoring are organised.

The limitations

The limitations to mentoring are perhaps best described by the use of the term toxic mentoring, identified by Darling (1986) and discussed earlier in this chapter. Toxic mentoring concerns the disabling elements and strategies that may be employed by an ineffective mentor and these should be avoided at all cost.

The essence of toxicity arises from a dysfunctional relationship that is not built on mutual trust, shared values or reciprocity. In a toxic rela-tionship the mentee is directed not facilitated, and ultimately disabled rather than enabled or supported. Toxic mentoring can take the form of an exploitative, manipulative relationship, the 'Queen bee, worker-drone syndrome' illustrated by Hawkins and Thibodeau (1989). The features of toxic mentoring are:

- The mentor uses the mentee and does not promote the mentee's ideas, taking any credit due
- Some recognition of a partnership but the mentor uses the mentee's abilities to further their own career and standing in the organisation
- The power in the relationship may remain with the mentor, resulting in mentee manipulation, over-protection, increased dependency, and lack of development
- Control and excessive direction causing the mentee to conform to an identical set image of the mentor, resulting in cloning
- Elitism and mutual seclusion causing the mentee to withdraw from other relationships and become dependent on the mentor.

Strategies for avoiding toxic mentors

(1) Self select a classical mentor or if offered a mentor programme, choose a mentor who is interested and who you can work with
(2) Do not choose an individual who is a disabler
(3) Examine the relationship regularly for signs of toxicity – cloning, dependency, mentor self-interest, manipulation or exploitation
(4) Monitor personal development and prepare a sound, appropriate end to the relationship
(5) Be prepared to eject from a mentor who is showing signs of toxi-city
(6) Ensure that the person chosen as a mentor is successful and 'going places' in the organisation.

Recognition of the benefits and limitations of mentoring facilitates a better understanding of what mentoring is all about and allows a healthy dialogue to commence regarding the salient issues that may arise.

Constraints to mentoring

Although personnel newly appointed to an organisation may have the necessary personal qualities for becoming a mentor, they are unlikely to have the networking contacts to provide for effective mentoring. As they settle to the organisation culture they will initially lack power, experience and possibly influence within the organisation. Research by Earnshaw (1995, p. 278) found stress was a problem for staff nurses who were expected to be mentors to students while they were 'trying to establish themselves professionally'.

Other constraints to effective mentoring – particularly classical mentoring – are working cultures where there is a rigid hierarchy or where disabling strategies prevail and there is subsequently a lack of collegiality and trust. Clutterbuck (1985) further identifies problems in organisations where heavy politics are evident, staff turnover is high and morale is poor, all acting as deterrents to effective mentoring.

Mentoring limitations of working cultures where women make up the majority of the workforce, and how this affects the existence of mentoring, are well documented by writers exploring the nature of mentoring May *et al.*, 1982, p.27; Hardy, 1984). It is important to note that in nursing, midwifery and other professional groups where the majority of the working population is female, there remain issues of gender and professional identification to be taken into account (Davies, 1995).

Women's working image and self-esteem along with the training and education of women in professional groups, and their socialisation into vocational work, have to be further explored and researched. Whilst there is evidence for constraints, such as women having to make it alone and having little time or effort left to support others, there is growing evidence that women do indeed identify with the need to support and bring others along as they make their way though corporate and professional environments, (Segerman-Peck, 1991; Conway, 1996).

Others suggest that women do help and support each other, even if they do not formally recognise this assistance as mentoring (Vance, 1979). Although not always recognising or fully appreciating the networking qualities of the processes involved, Sheehy (1976, p. 34), reported that 'women who haven't had a mentor relationship miss it, even if they don't know what to call it'. The confusion about mentoring over the years has added to the difficulties of role recognition and this comment could now apply equally well to men.

However, when considering women and mentoring, it is important to appreciate the issues of language, organisational context and sexual stereotyping in formulating, reflecting and reinforcing ideologies of gender (Demarco, 1993; Parsons, 1993). Formal mentoring programmes constructed from business orientated models may indeed offer a foundation for design but should be adapted to readily encompass the working needs of women in health care.

Contemplating such issues leads us to the need to consider the effective development and implementation of mentoring programmes that capture the richness of the relationship. It is now appropriate that we consider mentoring in action. The early part of this chapter focused particularly on the nature of the classical mentor and how this has been translated through history and by differing organisational challenges and demands. In considering the application of mentoring in practice it is necessary to contemplate the more structured systems and processes that exist in the form of formal or contract (facilitated) mentoring.

Formal mentoring: devising a mentor programme

In setting up a mentor programme, with the notion of providing formal or contract mentoring in the workplace with formal mentors or contract mentors, it is important to appreciate the complexities involved. Whether the decision is made to build your own programme or buy in a 'ready made, adapted to fit your needs programme' the groundwork has to be thorough and the intentions clear if the venture is to be a success. For diagrammatic representation of a workable model for practice see Fig. 2.3, which presents an overview; Fig. 2.4 illustrates the processes involved.

Design deliberations should include:

- The type of mentoring approaches to be employed
- Resource allocation
- Mentor-mentee preparation and support
- Effective evaluation.

Resources and approaches

Resources and approaches will depend on the requirements of the organisation, what is available and the commitment of senior staff for this type of support development. A general shift towards an appreciation that a learning culture is good for staff, customers and business has led to manufacturers providing increased resources for staff development (Ball,

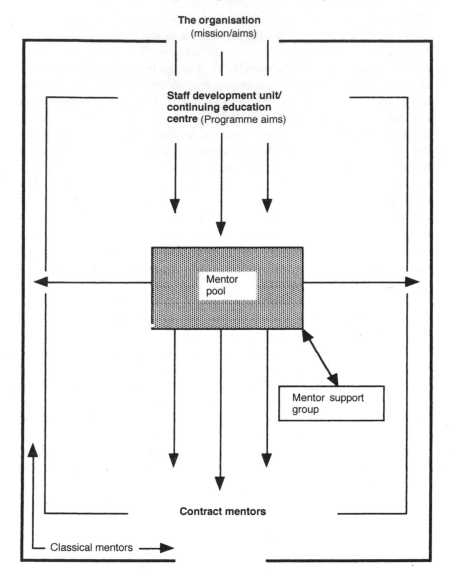

Fig. 2.3   Mentoring – an overview of a workable model in practice.

1992). Those interested in developing mentoring programmes within the health service can draw on the experiences of these other organisations to convince managers that effective investment in sound programmes will have an impact on staff with the ultimate aim of improving patient/client care. There is increasing evidence that mentoring is effective as part of a recognisable staff development programme and benefits working relationships (Kelly, 1992; Mumford, 1998).

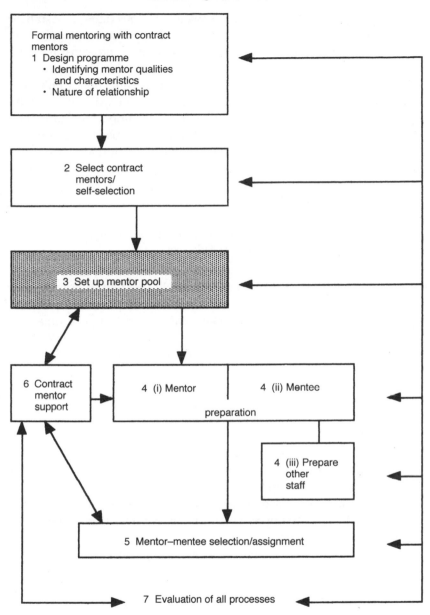

Fig. 2.4 A workable model for practice: processes involved.

Sensible resource decisions also require consideration of the types of approaches to be used. It is uneconomical to devise intricate formal mentoring structures with extensive mentor preparation if what is required is staff induction and orientation. Of course these elements can be incorporated into the contract mentoring role, but it will not be cost effective if the process required is someone to introduce new staff or acclimatise those who are returning to work. Practical induction and orientation processes can be readily incorporated into existing management roles.

Effective economies can be made by shared learning opportunities or by including mentor preparation in other programmes that focus on interpersonal, facilitation and enabling skills. Mentors, preceptors and clinical supervisors can be prepared together for part of a common programme, as long as the similar elements and differences are made very clear. This should work well in aiding understanding of each other's role. It will help to start the 'mutual respect and sharing philosophies' necessary to underpin such developments and to prevent the possibility of a 'hierarchy of roles' developing.

It is worth mentioning prepared mentor packages at this point as there are a variety of models available. We describe these as:

- *The Takeaway* – ready-made off the shelf; just add to your organisation or department
- *The Savile Row* – made-to-measure and tailored to your organisation's individual needs
- *The Pick and Mix* – selected from ready-made models and adapted to your individual preference.

When considering bought in, prepared or tailored mentoring packages there are important questions to consider:

(1) Are they flexible for the organisation's needs? Does the programme match with the mission, aims, philosophies, value systems and organisational culture?
(2) How are the mentors' roles and functions perceived? How does this fit in with existing support and development roles that already exist in the organisation?
(3) What are the cost implications of buying and then running the programme?
(4) Is programme evaluation included and how does it operate?
(5) Can a sound, cost-effective programme be prepared within the organisation or is consultation required?

Mentor–mentee preparation and support

This remains a developing area with the type, duration of preparation and resulting support networks for the mentors appearing as extremely varied. A range of formal programmes exists which can be seen to relate to a continuum, from those closely aligned to the characteristics of classical mentoring (Hernandez-Piloto Brito, 1992) to more formal functional structures where contracts are set and mentors assigned and monitored (Anworth, 1992) (see Fig. 2.5): the continuum of informality and formality. Preparing mentors remains a contentious subject and is an aspect of the process that would benefit from further research and perhaps case studies to illuminate the processes involved in adequate preparation. Fish (1995, p. 30), in identifying mentor education for what she calls 'quality' mentors in education, makes the point that preparation should include consideration of rights and responsibilities; awareness of partnership agreements and contractual obligations; and an understanding of articulating theory and practice, as well as the development of practice skills to assist the mentor with forming an effective relationship. She suggests that this gives the mentors a sense that they have a 'new competence'.

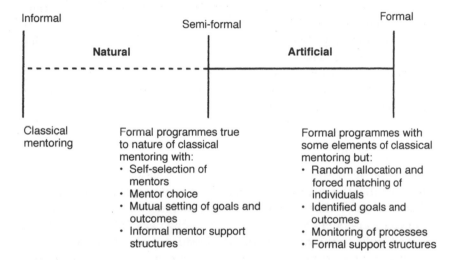

Fig. 2.5 Mentoring: the continuum of informality and formality.

In social work practice where mentoring is applied at the post qualifying level and is linked to the Advanced Award in Social Work, training for mentors is advocated and guidelines identified for the type of experience and qualifications required of those preparing for this essentially educational role. What separates this from other mentor training is the inclusion of the need to provide evidence from practice of anti-racist, anti-oppressive and anti-discriminatory practice. This goes further than other mentor programmes, where potential mentors have to demonstrate commitment to adult learning and continuing professional education, as well as capabilities of personal awareness, effective communication skills and sound abilities to relate to others.

The business organisation approach, where the mentor may have a more clearly defined role in relation to managing change and developing leaders and executives, offers useful case studies for mentor preparation. Slipais (1993) identifies a development process that combines in-house training, experience as an instructor, refresher sessions and formal advanced preparation which should include training skills, task analysis, communication skills, problem solving and decision-making (Slipais, 1993, pp. 134-5).

Other authors identify certificated preparation for mentorship and a variety of preparation approaches that range from the residential to day release or in-service programmes (Wilkin, 1992). In identifying a programme for preparing 'holistic mentors', Freeman (1998, p. 54) describes a scheme with introductory workshops to enable would be mentors 'to work freely and confidently at their task, maximising potential for their own professional task'. In preparing mentors using a collaborative learning approach, the GP mentors were encouraged through a series of reflective workshops to explore their understanding of role and develop effective enabling skills.

Despite the passing years and greater awareness of mentoring generally, the other main contentious issues remain those of mentor selection and mentor–mentee matching.

Mentor selection

As can be seen from the discussions on classical mentoring, it is important that the mentor is capable of the qualities, characteristics and skills inherent within an enabling role. Mentors are required to feel competent, confident and committed to taking part. Failures in the past of not building and maintaining relationships probably resulted from forced matching or random allocation of individual participants. This was true particularly, for example, in British nursing education, where staff irrespective of their experience or expertise were given mentoring responsibilities for a number of students at a time.

The statement 'appropriately qualified and experienced individual' appears to have become a popular way of identifying possible mentors and it is important to identify what is meant by such a broad statement. The term 'qualified' has formal and informal connotations in this context. It may be interpreted to mean that an individual has completed a recognisable training or education programme, or in its broadest sense it may relate to the capabilities of the mentor in terms of the personal qualities that they possess.

It is for the programme developers, educators, administrators and managers within a particular setting to clarify what is meant by 'appropriately qualified and experienced', and to state what they require from mentors. Clearly identified aims and a selected target audience for the preparation programme, with an appropriate definition of the characteristics and capabilities of the mentor, will assist successful implementation (Wilson, 1998).

The mentor pool

To assist in making informed selections a mentor pool may be needed and this should be identified early in the programme deliberations. A mentor pool is a group of people with appropriate qualities, abilities and experience to take on the rigours and complexities of mentoring. Ideally, this pool should consist of volunteers who are aware of the nature of mentoring (by personal experience or identified criteria), and who are prepared to become committed to a formal programme and its aims.

Setting identified criteria and 'trawling' for mentors can take a variety of forms: some programmes have involved marketing techniques (Hernandez-Piloto Brito, 1992); others ask for volunteers, or prospective mentors are chosen/volunteered by their managers. Being chosen or volunteered has potential drawbacks, minimised if consultation and negotiation take place between all those involved. Being volunteered for mentor selection particularly increases the risks of toxic mentoring, mismatching of individuals and personality clashes (Palmer, 1986).

Mentor–mentee matching

Mentor–mentee matching will remain contentious until there is sufficient evidence to demonstrate whether freedom to choose or forced matching of mentors provides the best method for assigning mentees. Access to a mentor pool allows individuals to make some form of selection, and this process is assisted if the members of the pool prepare brief mentor-biographies of professional and personal experiences. These identify their main interests, work experiences and the helper functions they can offer a potential mentee.

Time will need to be set aside within the programme for facilitated sessions where the mentors and mentees can meet for introductions, the sharing of relevant biographies and setting guidelines for the relationship. The informal meetings that arise from these initial discussions can then be left to the individuals concerned to arrange, supported if necessary by an identified mentor coordinator or facilitator.

Effective criteria, appropriate selection and time allocated for 'making the match' should ensure that freedom to choose does indeed occur. Issues of mentor–mentee ratios can tax the uninitiated; however, taking into consideration the time, effort and commitment required, it is suggested that a mentor should not have more than two mentees at any one time.

It is also important to build workshop sessions into a programme, to follow up on any mentors who may be disappointed in not being selected. This may be important with the development of such a new initiative and where mentors may well be selected or proposed by their managers. Until the parameters have been tested and flexibly set, it may be the case that people will be asked to attend a mentor course, by managers and administrators, in order to gain enabling skills – rather in the traditional manner of being sent on communication courses to learn how to communicate! It needs to be stressed to all concerned that this is not the aim of mentor programmes.

This should become less of a problem as mentoring becomes a better understood concept and as selection criteria are more adequately addressed. Complementary, enabling programmes can be devised and worked into a framework of continuing professional education that will feed into appropriate support role programmes to inform other staff who may be involved only indirectly.

The programme

The essence of mentor preparation involves an exploration of the nature of mentoring, the processes, benefits and limitations. Programme aims, strategies, content and outcomes will vary considerably depending on the needs of the organisation and the personnel involved. It is important that the programme has clear, well-defined outcomes as it should facilitate:

- An understanding of support within continuing professional development
- The clarification of new roles and support frameworks
- Opportunities to enhance enabling skills in relation to the helper functions
- Feedback on individual performance
- Opportunities for shared learning
- Networks of personal support and guidance
- Understanding of toxic strategies and possible role conflict
- An understanding of how mentoring fits within the organisation.

Many care workers and professionals in the health field already have preparation containing elements of this type of programme. What needs to be stressed, however, is the need to refocus on certain attitudes and skills to include coaching, consultation and feedback that may not be readily apparent in other continuing professional education pro-grammes. It is also crucial to the effectiveness of such a programme that the aims, teaching, facilitating and support strategies should be con-gruent with the open, enabling philosophy of this type of relationship. It is also important that programme aims or philosophies match those of the organisation, as previously discussed.

There is no universally agreed length of programme and some mentor preparation has been included in statutory teaching and assessing courses. This usually involves the allotment of two hours or an afternoon to discover the complexities of mentoring. Tuck (1993) very briefly outlines a two day training course for mentors and their 'clients' that relates reflective activities to curriculum skills and the interpersonal skills of mentoring. Other programmes have been devised to incorporate a series of workshop days to facilitate a better understanding; however, suggestions have been made that a basic training of five days is appro-priate to provide more time for the actual processes (Wright, 1990; Kelly *et al.*, 1991; Palmer, 1998).

Evidence has emerged regarding the implementation and evaluation of mentoring programmes and formal mentoring approaches based on assigning contract mentors. *The Mentor's Task: Main Activities and Standards*, prepared by the Oxford Brookes University and Oxford Health Authority, is documented in Heslop and Lathlean (1991, p.113).

An investigation into the development and running of an initial teacher training (ITT) course mentor programme is analysed by Corbett and Wright (1993). Their two year, school-based ITT programme involved asking head teachers to select a teacher to act as a mentor for those on the course. Mentors were offered financial reward and some freeing of their time by one half day per week supply cover. Certain issues surfaced as the study progressed, including:

- The crucial role of the head teacher in setting the mentor culture
- The teacher's development was linked to the development of the mentor
- Certain groups of individuals appeared better suited to provide the mentor role; these were identified as those new to teaching and those with more experience but with no senior management responsibilities
- Effective skills and approaches concerned areas of organisation, communication, counselling, supporting, monitoring, collaboration and problem solving
- A willingness to learn, develop and engage in learning were viewed as necessary attributes for mentor selection. Mentors needed to recognise change in their mentees, and to allow them to establish their own capabilities and responses

- Mentor training was found to be a restrictive term and mentor development better advised. Development should include broad range activities such as attending conferences, manager support, accredited study and informal mentor networks.

Respecting that it is not advisable to generalise from one study, it is interesting to note that this analysis goes some way towards validating previous deliberations. It offers evidence for the type of considerations and decisions to be made for those planning similar mentoring schemes. Regular follow-up sessions should be accommodated within each scheme to explore emerging issues as the mentoring relationships develop, and to provide support for each mentor.

Supporting the mentor

By providing effective preparation and in acknowledging the need for mentor support, mentors are able to make contact with each other and share the challenges that arise. Depending on the degree of formality of the structured programme on offer, they can build and develop their own networks. Highly experienced individuals of the calibre required to be effective mentors will already, as discussed earlier, have made themselves a niche in the organisation.

The need for recognisable and more structured methods of support for mentors has mainly arisen due to the indiscriminate use of this concept in some clinical areas. In classical mentoring, support should be negotiable and informal and the appropriate mechanisms developed by the mentors themselves. While formal mentoring may be more structured in approach, it is still the participating individuals who decide on the nature of the relationship and how it runs its course. This will allow them the freedom to identify and explore salient issues within a clear remit of respecting the confidentiality of the mentoring relationships.

Excessive formal structure with monitoring and feedback reflects traditional rigidity that is inappropriate for this type of enabling relationship or programme. Taking a rigid approach may deflect some of the intricate interactions from the mentor–mentee partnership and raise concerns regarding the maintenance of confidentiality and mutuality.

Evaluation

Evaluation plays an important part in professional practice and is an essential element in any new design process (Palmer & Wilson, 1997). Its importance in constructing formal mentoring programmes is significant because of the lack of empirical evidence and the confusion and contentious nature of the concept (McIntyre *et al.*, 1993; Maggs, 1994). Information obtained from sound evaluation techniques will aid future mentoring deliberations and developments.

A combination of quantitative and qualitative evaluation approaches is useful to illuminate the complexities of making formal programmes work in practice settings. Such studies should be set within the context of a realistic assessment of the resources available. This is elaborated by Puetz (1992) in her discussion of evaluation and staff development issues. A checklist for designing an evaluation of a programme has been formulated by Murray and Owen (1991, p. 172). In considering the appropriate approaches to be used, it is recommended that both the value to the individual and to the organisation should be included in any evaluation deliberations. For a very helpful discourse on evaluation and the issues that may arise, see Carter (1993).

A simple evaluative framework of reflective questions is identified in Chapter 4 for considering the effectiveness of the clinical supervision relationship within practice. A phased approach is suggested to uncover the processes, functions and roles involved and this could be easily adapted for evaluation of a mentoring relationship (see Chapter 4).

Whatever evaluation methods are decided on, it is a useful technique when exploring this complexity of the relationship to record the experiences of those involved, and this is where qualitative research approaches can be beneficial in further illuminating the mentoring relationship in depth. Collecting narratives and asking individuals to record their reactions, expectations and feelings can only further our understanding of what remains a fascinating relationship. As Demarco (1993) urges, we should become conscious of our biases towards this type of relationship and explore the 'lived experience'.

The case studies that follow are offered to add to the richness of the discussion and encourage further reflection about this significant professional support role.

Reflection: mentoring case studies

These case studies are not intended to be fully representative, but to provide an outline of different types of mentoring relationships. Indeed, in two of the studies presented concerns are raised and mentoring does not appear to have occurred in the richness that is so often reported. Many informal and formal mentoring relationships are positive and develop (through the stages identified previously in this chapter) to become very useful and enabling for those involved. Presenting these practical applications allows some of the issues surrounding mentoring in practice to be highlighted and reflected on.

As you read through the studies you might like to identify relevant issues that you feel are important in relation to what has been discussed in this chapter and your own experiences of mentoring. If you identify a significant relationship that had or has the elements of classical or contract mentoring, you could ask yourself the following questions, recording your deliberations in your portfolio/reflective journal or whatever you use to capture your experiences and reflections:

- What personal qualities did the person have that attracted you to him/ her?
- How did they help or support?
- Why did you want to work with, or learn from him/her?

Reflection: What is emerging from this information and how will it help you build significant relationships in the future?

The new community midwife nurse

Chris is a very experienced community midwife in her early 30s. She is keen, quick thinking and considered by those around her as a good manager, being well liked and respected by both peers and the women she is responsible for. She enjoys teaching and, 'seeing those around me settle in, obtain midwifery experience and get on'.

When Pauline, a new community midwife joins the district, Chris elects to orientate her and the two of them 'hit it off' immediately. Pauline is a mature woman who has returned to community midwifery, 'after taking time out to have the children'. Despite the obvious age gap, Chris senses 'something of myself' in Pauline's attitudes and responses to her work with the mothers and babies.

They get on well together during Pauline's orientation period, with Chris interested in sharing her experience of the busy district. When work loads and team commitments allow, the two spend time discussing their cases and experiences. Pauline is quick to learn, respects Chris' judgment and shows a willingness to become involved in all aspects of midwifery in the community. They remain good working companions and although Pauline appears eager to meet more often, they manage to meet only infrequently because of the changing nature of community care and differing shift patterns. Chris makes time but gradually meeting together becomes a rare event. Chris is disappointed that the opportunities to share good practice and discuss 'our ideas for the future of midwifery have become less and less, as we pass like two ships in the night'.

Newly qualified and moving on

Sue is 26 years old and a student midwife. Her most recent post was as a registered nurse on a renal surgical ward at the hospital that she trained in. As a third year she did well on this particular placement and found she liked and respected the ward sister, Carol Williams. On qualifying she asked to go back there to staff and 'to learn about looking after patients with renal problems and ward organisation'.

Sister Williams was much older than Sue and nearing retirement but had lost none of her keenness for caring for patients and making them comfortable in hospital. She was always the first to arrive on an early shift and the last to leave on a late one, despite having a family and social commitments. As Sue explains, 'She was part of the old school and I admired her for her personal abilities and nursing skills; she was always willing to share her experiences and spend time with me'. During the first year the sound, easy-going relationship continued. Sue was quick to learn and Sister Williams, whilst not singling her out from the other team members for extra support, encouraged and spent time with her. Sue felt trusted to 'run things when Sister wasn't there', and she grew in self-confidence and became more competent in her abilities to handle difficult situations.

Towards the end of the second year, Sue began to get restless as her friends and colleagues discussed different courses and plans for travelling. She shared her thoughts with Sister who had always been ready to listen and counsel in the past. However it was different this time and 'I soon became aware that she didn't want to know about me moving on or doing my midwifery which is what I had always planned to do'. Sue went ahead and applied and was accepted for a midwifery programme in the autumn. She was unprepared for Sister's negative response to the news, and despite maintaining a semblance of cordiality whilst working together for the remainder of her notice, Sue and Sister never really spoke again. Sue left the ward without saying goodbye, 'as Sister changed her day off and didn't attend my leaving party'.

Mature and keen to care

Peter is a physiotherapy student. He has had numerous jobs and spent the last few years as an air traffic controller. He decided to become a physiotherapist after caring for a relation following a road traffic accident. He is one of only three mature students on his course and the only male student. He is enjoying the course and gets on well with his peers, although he sometimes gets 'frustrated by their lack of life experience and flippant attitudes to serious concerns'. He is doing well academically and as the course has a formal mentor scheme he is assigned a mentor for his first clinical placement, which he is looking forward to.

Elizabeth is a bright, articulate, eager to teach individual who is younger than Peter. She volunteered for the hospital mentor scheme and enjoys 'the one-to-one relationship with a colleague, teaching and advising them and seeing them develop as they come to terms with what is expected of them as a student and finally a qualified physiotherapist'. Initially Peter and Elizabeth appear to 'hit it off', but gradually Elizabeth becomes aware that Peter does not readily seek her company. He appears to meet with her reluctantly, and only when she suggests they get together to discuss his progress in the clinical placements and on the course. Over several months, with little progress in the relationship and tensions on both sides, Peter asks his personal tutor if he can change mentors and choose his own this time.

The teacher and mentoring comparisons

Amy is a teacher and she has had 'two significant mentoring relationships', as she puts it, in her career as a teacher. She is currently a faculty head in a department for children with special needs, having moved from Expressive Arts recently. When she started as a young teacher she formed a mutually supportive relationship with the head of her department. They got on well, sharing the same views on teaching and had a similar sense of humour. They worked very well together and Amy found that Jan helped her settle into her new teaching role, as well as helping her to learn about how the school worked. In the early stages of the relationship Amy found that she relied on Jan for her considerable expertise and extensive knowledge. In return Amy would share her ideas and was happy to take on the projects that Jan put her way.

When Jan left to take up a senior teacher's post in a neighbouring community college, it was mutually agreed that Amy would move to the same college as there was a vacant post at a higher incentive allowance. To Amy it seemed 'a sensible option and there was also the possibility of promotion and of course Jan was going too'. After a successful interview, Amy joined the Expressive Arts Faculty.

In the new college Amy settled in well and her relationship with Jan 'continued much as before'. However after several months Amy became aware that Jan, who initially shared ideas and appeared keen to promote their joint work and projects, was changing. In the new setting Jan 'was now taking my ideas and putting them forward as her own; she even presented a paper at an INSET day that I had written, without acknowledging me. I felt I was doing all the hard work, but kept in the background'. Amy attempted to talk this over with Jan with little effect.

Amy left to head a faculty in a different school at the beginning of the new term. She now feels settled and is experiencing a much more positive working relationship with a deputy head, that is supportive and enabling. 'I feel I'm developing in an equal power relationship, able to be me and getting credited with what I do best.' She feels she can be creative, share her ideas and has something to offer her new mentor and faculty.

Classical mentoring: positive returns

Karen was a young occupational therapist when she first joined the faculty of health sciences at a new London University. She had always enjoyed the clinical aspects of occupational therapy (OT) but had always been drawn to teaching, 'interested in sharing her knowledge and clinical expertise'. She completed a postgraduate certificate in education at the university and then joined the staff, as a lecturer. Karen is an outgoing, affable person who has a keen sense of fun and a deep commitment to her chosen profession.

Following the first year in her lecturing post she remained undecided about a career in higher education and felt 'the loss of my clinical identity; I missed the patients, clients and team work'. She found working with the students rewarding but experienced difficulties in settling into what was a 'rather traditional department with old fashioned approaches to teaching and learning at a time when educational methods were advancing'.

Karen's attempts at introducing problem-based learning to one of her courses were met with resistance by other members of the department. She was feeling unsettled when a chance, informal meeting with the head of the department, Edwina, altered her perspective. Edwina was a visionary, extremely capable with an encouraging, honest manner and she did not take herself too seriously despite her position and stature in the OT world. Edwina spoke of the changes and the dilemmas that were occurring as new approaches and methods were considered in OT. She spoke of her commitment to developing education initiatives that would benefit the students and their patients and assist staff to come to terms with the challenges in education and health. This 'sounded like a blueprint for a better future and I could identify with that', Karen remembers afterwards.

Following their initial meeting Edwina invited Karen to join a faculty working party to develop a new curriculum. Over a period Karen found herself more and more involved in the affairs of the department and taking increasing responsibility for new projects. This led to more settled feelings and 'a renewed sense of purpose; I felt as if a new wider world had opened up and I felt very much a part of it'.

The relationship with Edwina was developing positively and Karen found she could discuss issues with her and on the occasions ' when I put my foot in it and got things wrong, I was assisted to see the error of my ways without being made to feel insignificant; I could be creative and take some risks but as time went on the risks and mistakes reduced as Edwina and I became tuned in'. When the principal lecturer's post was advertised Karen felt confident to apply and despite strong external opposition, impressed the panel with her abilities.

Following this senior appointment she found herself working more closely with Edwina, observing her style of management and leadership qualities at first hand. As their relationship developed, and was openly acknowledged as that of classical mentoring, Karen began to specifically choose the assistance she needed. 'At first I wanted anything Edwina had to offer, it was exciting and stimulating, but as time went on I felt confident to make choices. I asked to be sponsored for a course and I began to know instinctively when I needed counselling or just wanted advice.' With Edwina's support, Karen joined the College of OT as a regional council member. She began to play a part in

exploring wider concerns of the profession: 'Edwina opened up a new world to me by asking me to join committees and ultimately, as our respect and trust grew, I began to take her place at certain meetings.' Karen found that they worked out ideas together in a relationship where challenges and tensions could be met head on and strategies devised for success.

After seven years Karen knew it was time to move on: 'I felt capable of taking a leadership role for myself.' Together they explored the possibilities of future job prospects and Karen felt that at the start Edwina was rather reticent at the thought of her moving on: 'She would mention a post, leave the job description on my desk and say don't think about it too long'. Talking over the proposed move together made it more real and Karen's reflections of this period suggest that it was a time of excitement at the prospects of new horizons but sadness as a chapter closed in her working life. 'I felt I was getting ahead now and Edwina admitted that sometimes she felt she was following in my footprints instead of leading the way'.

Finally, after Edwina and Karen discovered the same post in separate advertisements, they knew this was the time to move on. Karen successfully applied for the head of school's post at a northern university, She is now a nationally respected figure representing OT at the highest levels. Edwina has now retired but they remain in regular contact and have become firm friends who still like nothing better than 'getting together to discuss OT issues and the changes that lie ahead'.

Case studies: the issues

Sue and Sister Williams built up a good relationship that started when Sue went originally to the ward in her final year of her education programme. They had a mutual interest in their chosen speciality and common commitments to patient care and ward management. What starts for Sue as admiration and role modelling is extended to a more rounded, enabling relationship as Sister gives time to her and shares her clinical expertise. Sue is willing to learn and with her motivation and interest in the ward, she becomes a worthwhile partner in caring for the patients. It is readily apparent that mutual admiration and respect has developed.

Problems occur when Sue wishes to move on. Sister is possessive and not ready to let go. She is nearing retirement and possibly fears the changes that will result when Sue leaves. She has also invested time and effort into the relationship, and careful negotiation and a gradual separation are required in this type of situation. Although it may appear in classical mentoring, mentor possessiveness is a more common criticism offered by mentees in more formal mentoring programmes. Feelings of being trapped can occur when the mentee is submissive and unable to remove themselves from what they see as a claustrophobic situation. In both types of mentoring, making both individuals fully aware of the processes and phases of mentoring can go some way towards preventing this difficulty and allowing endings to be more positive. As it is, Sue was unable to resolve the situation and was unprepared for Sister William's distancing behaviour; the relationship ends negatively without the rewards of maintaining contact and friendship.

Pauline is returning to midwifery in the community and although having to face new challenges she is a mature individual. She may well know her own mind at this time of her life or indeed may not recognise the need for support at this stage. Chris and Pauline are mutually attracted, and seemingly get on and work well together. Chris is apparently sending out mentor signals but these are not being picked up by Pauline as she settles into the rigours of busy midwifery life. Work commitments, lack of regular contact and different shift systems are inhibiting the natural processes of mentoring. Although Chris has been helpful in orientating Pauline and assisting her to settle in her new post, there is no time to build on the mutual attraction and respect that has initially occurred. Chris appears ready to mentor and it is highly probable that she will continue to send out signals that will be eventually taken up when an appropriate individual and right circumstances prevail.

Peter is a mature student and has been assigned a mentor, in this case a younger female who is keen to help him in his first placement. Peter may be well aware of his needs and we do not know how he has been prepared for the mentoring experience. Sound preparation, with time allotted to get properly acquainted, assist potential mentees to set realistic expectations.

Peter's case raises issues of cross-gender mentoring and although not identified in this chapter, there are other implications when contract mentoring involves individuals from differing cultures and ethnic groups. Cross-gender mentoring is extensively covered in business and can be associated with sexual liaisons either actual or implied by others, who may well be motivated by favouritism or jealousy. The possibility of sexual tensions and attractions between individuals of different or the same sex should be acknowledged in initial mentor orientation, and the outcomes and complications discussed openly.

Risks of personality clashes can occur when mentors are assigned and a mismatch of personalities occurs. From the author's own research and personal experience, if an assigned mentor is not seen to be meeting the needs of the assigned mentee and if there is any dissatisfaction or hostility, then the mentee will seek a more appropriate individual and set up informal mentoring networks elsewhere. These often run parallel to those planned and directed by the staff educators. We do not know what preparation Peter has had or his expectations for this type of relationship, but he draws our attention to issues of choice in selecting a mentor. It is also important to consider Elizabeth's preparation and experience of mentoring; she may have only been assigned younger or female students previously.

Amy and Jan's case illustrates potential power relationships in mentoring which may evoke similar reactions and endings to those between Sue and Sister Williams. In this situation, Jan with her charisma and winning ways could be seen as enticing the initially submissive Amy. In negative terms, Jan is using her to further her own development and career. Mutuality has ceased and the power balance has shifted towards that of meeting the needs of a powerful, controlling mentor.

Amy, in changing jobs, moves the focus from that of her own needs and development to that of maintaining Jan's credibility in the new college. This study presents us with an example of the 'queen bee/worker drone syndrome': if one party remains submissive and readily supplies the 'queen bee', the two can advance through the hierarchy together until circumstances cause them to fall out or drift apart. In this example, Amy is able to recognise what is happening and is very capable in acting quickly to get herself out of the situation. She is then able to commence a new relationship with the deputy head in the new college. This relationship is much more aligned to that of true classical mentoring. Amy experiences none of the toxicity of the previous encounter and is able to feel confident in sharing in more collaborative surroundings.

The last case demonstrates the positive aspects of classical mentoring in terms of the natural nature of the collaboration – the mutual rewards and the longevity as the two individuals start to trust, share and respect each other. This is similar in essence to the supportive and enabling relationship that Amy, in the previous case, has begun at her new school. Karen's commitment and need for change are recognised by her senior colleague. A relationship develops that assists Karen to sort out her feelings about her career, to become involved in departmental initiatives and to rehearse areas of learning that facilitate an awareness of her own abilities.

In the early stages of the relationship Karen notes the need for any type of support and is not discerning in selecting what she requires. However, as the mutual trust, honesty, communication and respect build, she becomes more confident to choose the assistance she requires. Karen is well aware of the risks she takes and the development that occurs. The personal guidance offered is such that she maintains her self-esteem and confidence, as well as being encouraged to learn from less positive events. Karen is able to develop her own professional identity constructively, eventually leading to her taking a significant leadership role in her chosen profession. Edwina in her retirement, can feel satisfied that she played a part in Karen's success and that she has left her profession in capable hands.

These cases have demonstrated a range of issues and I am sure that you will have identified others within the examples given and from contemplation of your own experiences. It is only by illuminating mentoring in its many forms and by understanding how it works in practice, that we will be able to provide adequate programmes of preparation in the future. A clearer understanding of this intriguing subject will go some way towards removing the scepticism and negative effects that may arise from using the concept inappropriately and with little thought. Effective programmes and better understanding will also assist in encouraging those qualified practitioners wanting to become mentors to view mentoring as a recognition of their qualities, approachability and professionalism and not as a 'right'.

References

Alliott, R.J. (1966) Facilitating mentoring in general practice. *British Medical Journal*. Career focus series. 28 September, 1996.

Anworth, P. (1992) Mentors, not assessors. *Nurse Education Today*, **12** (4) 299–302.

Anderson, E.M. & Shannon, A.L. (1995) Towards a conceptualization of mentoring. In: T. Kerry and A.S. Shelton Mayes (eds) *Issues in Mentoring*, Routledge, London.

Armitage, P. & Burnard, P. (1991) Mentors or Preceptors? Narrowing the theory–practice gap. *Nurse Education Today*, **11** (3) 225–9.

Ashton, P. & Richardson, G. (1992) Preceptorship and PREPP. *British Journal of Nursing*, **1** (3), 143–6.

Ball, C. (1992) The learning society. *Royal Society of Arts Journal*, May, 380–94.

Barlow, S. (1991) Impossible dream. *Nursing Times*, **87**, 1:53–54.

Blotnick, S.R. (1984) With friends like these. *Savvy*, 10, 45–52.

Bould, J. (1996) *Getting it Right: Mentoring in Medicine. The Practical Guide.* University of Leeds. CCDU, Training & Consultancy.

Boydell, D. (1994) Relationships and feelings: the affective dimension to mentoring in primary school. *Mentoring and Tutoring*, **2** (2), 37–44.

Boydell, D. & Bines, H. (1994) Beginning teaching: the role of the mentor. *Education*, **22**, 29–33.

Brooks, V. & Sikes, P. (1997) *The Good Mentor Guide. Initial Teacher Education in Secondary Schools.* Open University Press, Buckingham.

Burnard, P. (1988) Self evaluation methods in nurse education. *Nurse Education Today*, **8**, 229–33.

Calkins, E.V., Arnold, L.M. & Willoughby, T.L (1987) Perceptions of the role of a faculty supervisor or 'mentor' at two medical schools. *Assessment and Evaluation in Higher Education*, **12** (3), 202–8.

Campbell-Heider, N. (1986) Do nurses need mentors? *IMAGE: Journal of Nursing Scholarship*, **18** (3), 110–13.

Cantor, L.M. & Roberts, I.F. (1986) *Further Education Today. A critical review*, 3rd edn. Routledge Kegan Paul, London.

Carter, E.M.A (1993) Measuring the returns. In: (eds B.J. Coldwell & E.M.A. Carter) *The Return of the Mentor. Strategies for workplace learning*. The Falmer Press, London.

CCETSW (1992) *The Requirements for Post Qualifying Education & Training in the Personal Social Services: A Framework for Continuing Professional Development*. Paper 31 revised education. Central Council for Education & Training in Social Work, London.

Clutterbuck, D. (1985) *Everybody Needs A Mentor – How To Further Talent Within An Organisation*. The Institute of Personnel Management, London.

Collins, E.G.C. & Scott, P. (1978) Everybody who makes it has a mentor. *Harvard Business Review*, July/August, 89–102.

Community Care (1998) Social exclusion – stand by me. *Community Care*, 29 January–4 February, 18–19.

Conway, C. (1996) Strategic role of mentoring. *Professional Manager, September, 1996*.

Cooper, M.D. (1990) Mentorship: the key to the future of professionalism in nursing. *Journal of Perinatal Neonatal Nursing*, **4** (3) 71–7.

Corbett, P. & Wright, D. (1993) Issues in the selection and training of mentors for school-based primary teacher training. In: *Mentoring: Perspectives on School-based Teacher Education*. (Eds D. McIntyre, H. Hagger & M. Wilkin), pp. 220–33. Kogan Page, London.

Cray, D. & Mallory, G.R. (1998) *Making Sense of Managing Culture*. Thomson Business Press, London.

Darling, L.A.W. (1984) What do nurses want in a mentor? *Journal of Nursing Administration*, **14** (10), 42–4.

Darling, L.A.W. (1986) What to do about toxic mentors. *Nurse Educator*, **11** (2), 29–30.

Davies, C. (1995) *Gender and the Professional Predicament in Nursing*. Open University Press, Buckingham.

Demarco, R. (1993) Mentorship: a feminist critique of current research. *Journal of Advanced Nursing*, **18** (1), 1242–50.

Department for Education (1992) *New Criteria and Proceeds for Accreditation of Courses of Initial Teacher Training*. Circular 9/92. HMSO, London.

DoH, (1997) *The New NHS: Modern – Dependable*. Department of Health, London.

Earnshaw, G.J. (1995) Mentorship: the studentís views. *Nurse Education Today*, 15, 274–9.

ENB (1987) *Institutional and Course Approval/Reapproval Process, Information Required – Criteria and Guidelines*, 1987/28/MAT. English National Board, London.

ENB (1988) *Institutional and course approval/Reapproval Process, Information Required – Criteria and Guidelines*. 1988/39/APS. English National Board, London.

Eng, S.P. (1986) Mentoring in principalship education. In (Owen, M.A. & Murray, M) *Beyond the myths and magic of mentoring. How to facilitate an effective mentor program*, Jossey-Bass, Oxford.

Fagan, M.M. & Walter, G. (1982) Mentoring Among Teachers. *Journal of Educational Research*, **76** (2), 113–18.

Fields, W.L. (1991) Mentoring in Nursing: a Historical Approach. *Nursing Outlook*, Nov/Dec, 257–61.

Fish, D. (1995) *Quality Mentoring for Student Teachers. A principled approach to practice*. D. Fullan Publishers, London.

Freeman, R. (1997) Mentoring in General Practice. *Education for General Practice*, 7, 112–17.

Freeman, R. (1998) *Mentoring in GP Practice*. Heinneman Butterworth, London.

George, P. & Kummerow, J. (1981) Mentoring for career women. *Training*, **18** (2), 44, 46–9.

Glover, D., Gough, G., Johnson, M., Mardle, G. & Taylor, M. (1994) Towards a taxonomy of mentoring. *Mentoring and Tutoring*, **2** (2), 25–30.

Hagerty, B. (1986) A second look at mentors: do you really need one to succeed in nursing? *Nursing Outlook*, **34** (1), 16–19, 24.

Hamilton, M.S. (1981) Mentorhood, a key to nursing leadership. *Nursing Leadership*, **4** (1), 4–13.

Handy, C. (1985) *Understanding Organisations*. Penguin Business, Harmondsworth.

Hardy, L.K. (1984) The emergence of nurse leaders: in case of, in spite of, not because of. *International Nursing Review*, **31** (1), 11–15.

Hawkins, J.W. & Thibodeau, J.A. (1989) *The Nurse Practitioner and Clinical Nurse Specialist. Current Practice Issues*, 2nd edn. The Tiresias Press Inc., New York.

Hawkins, P. & Shohet, R. (1989) *Supervision in the helping professions*. Open University Press, Buckingham.

Heirs, B. & Farrell, P. (1986) *The Professional Decision Thinker – Our New Management Priority*, 2nd edn. Garden City Press Ltd, Hertfordshire.

Hernandez-Pilot Brito, H. (1992) Nurses in action. An innovative approach to mentoring. *Journal of Nursing Administration*, **22** (5), 23–8.

Heslop, A. & Lathlean, J. (1991) Teaching and learning, In: *Becoming a Staff Nurse – A guide to the role of the newly registered nurse*, (eds J. Lathlean & J. Corner. Prentice Hall, London.

Holloran, S. D. (1993) mentoring. The Experience of Nursing Service Executives. *Journal of Advanced Nursing*, **23** (2), 49–54.

Holloway, A. & Whyte, C. (1994) *Mentoring: The definitive handbook*. Development Processes (Publications) Ltd/Swansea College, Swansea.

Holt, R. (1982) An alternative to mentorship. *Adult education*, **55** (2), 152–6.

Hunt, D. & Michael, C. (1983) Mentorship. A career training development tool. *Academy of Management Review*, 3, 475–85.

James Report (1972) *Teacher Education and Training*. HMSO, London.

Jarvis, P. & Gibson, S. (1997) The Teacher-practitioner and Mentor in Nursing, Midwifery, Health Visiting and Social Services. Stanley Thornes, Cheltenham.

Kelly, K.J. (1992) *Nursing Staff Development. Current Competence Future Focus*. J.B. Lippincott, Philadelphia.

Kelly, M., Beck, T. & Thomas, J. (1991) More than a supporting act. *The Times Educational Supplement*, 8 November, 1991.

Klopf, G.J. & Harrison, J. (1981) Moving up the career ladder, the case for mentors. *Principal*, **61** (1), 41–3.

Knowles, MS. (1984) *Andragogy in Action: Applying Modern Principles of Adult Learning*. Jossey-Bass, San Francisco.

Kolb, D. A. (1984) *Experiential Learning*. Prentice Hall, New Jersey.

Levinson, D.J. Darrow, C.N., Klein, D.B., Levinson, M.H. & McKee, B. (1978) *The Season's of a Man's Life*. Knopf, New York.

MacPherson, H. (1997) Great talents ripen late. Continuing education in the acupuncture profession. *The European Journal of Oriental Medicine*, **1** (6), 35–9.

McIntyre, D. (1994) Classrooms as learning environments for beginning teachers. In: eds M. Wilkin & D. Sankey. Collaboration and Transition in Initial Teacher Training, Kogan Page, London.

McIntyre, D., Hagger, H. & Wilkin, M. (1993) *Mentoring. Perspectives on School-based Teacher Education*. Kogan Page, London.

Maggs, C. (1994) Mentorship in nursing and midwifery education: issues for research. *Nurse Education Today*, 14, 22–9.

May, K.M., Meleis, A.I. & Winstead-Fry, P. (1982) Mentorship for scholarliness, opportunities and dilemmas. *Nursing Outlook*, 30, Jan, 22–8.

Merriam, S. (1993) Mentors and proteges; a critical review of the literature. *Adult Education Quarterly*, **33** (3), 161–73.

Monaghan, J. & Lunt, N. (1992) Mentoring: person, process, practice and problems. *The British Journal Of Educational Studies*, **xxxx** (3), 239–47.

Morle, K.M.F. (1990) Mentorship, is it a case of the emperor's new clothes or a rose by any other name. *Nurse Education Today*, **10** (1), 66–9.

Morley, L. (1995) Theorising empowerment in the UK public services. *Empowerment in Organisations*, **3** (3) 35–41.

Muller, S. (1984) Physicians for the 21st century. Report of the project panel on general professional education of the physician's preparation for medicine. *Journal of Medical Education*, **59**, 2.

Mumford, A. (1998) Choosing Development Methods. *Organisations & People*, **5** (2), 32–7.

Murray, M. & Owen, M. A. (1991) *Beyond the Myths and Magic of Mentoring. How to Facilitate an Effective Mentor program*. Jossey-Bass, Oxford.

O'Hear, A. (1988) *Who Teaches the Teachers?* Social Affairs Unit, London.

Palmer, E. A (1987) *The nature of the mentor.* Unpublished thesis, South Bank Polytechnic.

Palmer, A. (1986) *Evaluation notes II for enrolled nurse conversion.* Unpublished project report, St. Mary's School of Nursing, London.

Palmer, A. (1992) *The role of the mentor in critical care.* Conference Paper, 7th Annual Conference, The British Association of Critical Care Nurses, September, Manchester University.

Palmer, A. (1998) *GP Mentoring and Practice Development.* London Inner Zone Education initiative, Academic Support Plan, Centre for Community Care and Primary Health, University of Westminster.

Palmer, A. & Wilson, A. (1997) *The Evaluation of 'Innovative Practice Projects'.* An evaluative study of 125 projects implemented within 34 NHS Trusts to support the 'New Deal' objectives. South Thames NHS Executive, London.

Parsloe, E. (1995) *Coaching, Mentoring and Assessing. A practical Guide to Developing Competencies*, revised edition. Kogan Page, London.

Parsons, S.F. (1993) Feminist challenges to curriculum design. In: *Culture and Processes of Adult Learning* (eds M. Thorpe, R. Edwardes & A. Hanson). Routledge, London.

Pelletier, D. & Duffield, C. (1994) Is there enough mentoring in nursing? *Australian Journal of Advanced Nursing*, **11** (4), 6–11.

Playdon, Z. (1998) Mentor the myth. In: *An Enquiry into Mentoring. Supporting Doctors and Dentists at Work*, Annex 3, Appendix 1, 32–5. SCOPME, London.

Pratt, J.W. (1989) Towards a philosophy of physiotherapy. *Physiotherapy*, **75** (2), 114–20.

Puetz, B.E. (1985) Learn the ropes from a mentor. *Nursing Success Today*, **2** (6), 11–13.

Puetz, B.E. (1992) Evaluation: Essential skill for the staff development specialists. In: *Nursing Staff Development: Current Competence, Future Focus*, (ed. K.J. Kelly), pp. 183–201. J. B. Lippincott Company, Philadelphia.

Raichura, L. & Riley, M. (1985) Introducing nurse preceptors. *Nursing Times*, 20 November, 40–42.

Roche, G.R. (1979) Much ado about mentors. *Harvard Business Review*, **56**, Jan/Feb, 14–18.

Rogers, C. (1983) *Freedom to Learn for the Eighties*, Charles E. Merrill, Columbus, Ohio.

Rumsey, H. (1995) *Mentors in Post Qualifying Education. An Interprofessional Perspective.* CCETSW, London.

Safire, W. (1980) On language. *New York Times Magazine*, Nov, 1980. Reported in: Mentoring for career women, (J. Kummerow & P. George) *Training*, **18** (2), 44, 46–9.

Sands, R. G., Parsons, L.A. & Duane, J. (1991) Faculty mentoring faculty in a public university. *Journal of Higher Education*, **62** (2), 175–93.

Schon, D. (1988) *Educating the Reflective Practitioner: Towards a New Design for Teaching and Learning in the Professions.* Jossey-Bass, London.

SCOPME, (1997) *Multiprofessional Working and Learning: Sharing the Educational Challenge*. Standing Committee on Postgraduate Medical & Dental Education, London.

SCOPME, (1998) *An Enquiry into Mentoring. Supporting Doctors and Dentists at Work*. Standing Committee on Postgraduate Medical & Dental Education, London.

Segerman-Peck, L. (1991) *Networking & Mentoring*. Judy Piatkus Publishers Ltd, London.

Sheehy, G. (1976) The mentor connection and the secret link in the successful woman's life. *New York Magazine*, **8**, 33–9.

Slipais, S. (1993) Coaching in a competency-based training system: The experience of the power brewing company. In: *The Return of the Mentor. Strategies for Workplace Learning*, (E.M.A. Carter, & B.J. Caldwell). The Falmer Press, London.

Smith, P. & West-Burnham, J. (1993) *Mentoring in the Effective School*. Longman Group UK, Essex.

Tomlinson, P. (1995) *Understanding Mentoring. Reflective Strategies for School-based Teacher Preparation*. Open University Press, Buckingham.

Tuck, R (1993) The Nature of Mentoring. *The New Academic*, Autumn, 25–6.

UKCC (1995) *PREP and You: Maintaining your Registration, Standards for Education Following Registration*, pp. 183–201. UKCC, London.

Vance, C.N. (1979) Women leaders: modern day heroines or societal deviants? *IMAGE, Journal of Nursing Scholarship*, **11** (2), 40–41.

Vance, C. (1982) The mentor connection. *The Journal Of Nursing Administration*, **12** (4), 7–13.

Weightman, J. (1996) *Managing People in the Health Service*. Institute of Personnel and Development. Cromwell Press, Wiltshire.

Weil, S. (1992) Learning to change. In: *Managing fundamental change: shaping new purposes and roles in public services*. Report of a one day conference organised by the Office for Public Management, June 1992.

Wheatley, M. & Hirsch, M.S. (1984) Five ways to leave your mentor. *MS Magazine*, Sept, 106–8.

Wilkin, M. (ed) (1992) *Mentoring in Schools*. Kogan Page, London.

Wilson, A. (1998) *An Evaluation of the London Inner Zone Education Projects*. Centre for Community Care & Primary Health, University of Westminster.

Wright, C.M. (1990) An innovation in a diploma programme: the future potential of mentorship in nursing. *Nurse Education Today*, **10**, 355–9.

Zaleznik, A. (1977) Manager leaders, are they different? *Harvard Business Review*, **55** (3), 67–78.

Zey, M.G. (1984) *The Mentor Connection*. Dow Jones Irwin, Homewood Illinois.

Chapter 3
Becoming Accountable: Preceptorship in Clinical Practice

Introduction

The transition from student to newly qualified and accountable practitioner is a time of anxiety and uncertainty, while at the same time being the longed for goal of every student. Ever since the ground-breaking work of Benner & Benner (1979) and Kramer (1974) which gave the name '*reality shock*' to the phenomenon of disorientation experienced by the newly qualified, various attempts have been made to manage career transitions more effectively.

Twenty years later, however, calls were still being made for stakeholders to undertake more research into transitional learning, and preceptorship in particular, so that a better understanding of the relevance of education to the newly qualified may inform educational and professional learning support initiatives (Bain, 1996; Kapborg & Fischbein, 1998).

In the first edition of this book, we challenged readers to assess the potential for professional learning support systems in their own fields of practice. We argued then that the priorities for implementing support were:

- Establishing the policy and procedural steps necessary for the appraisal of existing support systems
- Establishing a basis for partnership with service and education colleagues
- Re-affirming the trust and respect offered to and between colleagues in the work situation
- Providing a forum for support which allows for uncertainties to be expressed calmly and clearly
- Accepting the need to explore mutual understanding of support roles and to clarify these for any future use.

prepare fledgling practitioners for the
and to help protect the public from the
ning practitioners has, however, been
K literature, most visibly by the demands
plementing clinical supervision to govern-
ot to downplay the importance of integrating
sion initiatives within existing professional
ect dealt with in detail in the next chapter of this
s a partial explanation of the reasons why pre-
ed comparatively little attention in the health care
educ   since 1993.

Most o1 .   rature that has been published refers to the North
American and antipodean models of preceptorship, most of which
concern the precepting of students in pre-registration education rather
than newly qualified practitioners and returners to nursing, midwifery
and health visiting, as is the official policy here in the UK (UKCC, 1993).
Theories of preceptorship which could apply usefully to both pre and
post-registration models of transitional learning support are still much in
demand.

As authors, we also set ourselves a challenge six years ago when we
said we would continue to stimulate and share in the debate over the
provision of meaningful professional support systems, a challenge that
has been put to the test by the enthusiasm and integrity of staff
attempting to build systems which reflect their own philosophies of
learning and ethical practice around the country. As Bain has pointed
out, however, the empirical evidence addressing preceptorship has
remained contradictory and inconsistent. Without additional substantive
evidence to demonstrate the effectiveness of preceptorship programmes
there is a real danger that they will be reduced to becoming condensed
orientation programmes or crash courses for survival (Bain, 1996) rather
than an effective preparation for practice as others have claimed (e.g.
Boyle *et al.*, 1997).

Clarification of the preceptor role is still an ambition to be realised
within the UK context, with some writers calling for the development of
a standardised approach as a way of dealing with the confusion
experienced by practitioners in planning for and managing preceptorship programmes:

'Adequate preparation for preceptorship can hardly be provided
while ambiguity over the role remains. There is an urgent need to
clarify what is expected of preceptors to enable adequate development of the role to be undertaken ... The role of preceptors
must be clarified to enable their functions to be clearly under-

stood and supported ... The potential for a first class system of nurse education exists and it is important that problems are addressed before the positive views of preceptorship diminish.'

(Coates & Gormley, 1997, p. 97)

Although articles about preceptorships appear sporadically in the nursing and medical education literature, their use does not seem to have filtered significantly into the professional therapies. The availability of preceptor support for the management of career transitions across professional, organisational and hierarchical boundaries has not yet been fully explored, despite clear potential for its use.

This chapter hopes to redress some of the balance in terms of the problems highlighted. It was our ambition when we wrote the first edition in 1993 to find out whether preceptorship offered tangible and visible rewards in terms of better retention and recruitment of staff, higher morale, and an increased sense of purpose and mission in improving the quality of care provided to patients and clients. The formulation of soundly researched models of good practice was our long-term aim.

Although this reads as something of a 'wish list' as regards being a realistic goal, the first and most obvious thing to do was to undertake research into preceptorship which would help us to construct a meaningful and authentic account of beginning practice in nursing. This might then help us to identify key areas for clarification and development across both our own and other disciplines and specialist areas of practice. What had been missing, we reasoned, was an empirical basis from which to generate ideas about preceptorship and to experiment with different strategies which might illuminate the preceptorship concept for us. We also wanted to help colleagues in the difficult business of setting up and maintaining a professional support system which would assist the newly qualified (and new in post) to meet the demands of demands of their profession and their roles as employees working within widely diverse institutions and workplaces. Such research would have to be manageable, affordable and carefully planned so as to take account of the possibilities, opportunities and constraints such fieldwork would provide.

The *outcomes* of the collaborative research undertaken by the author – a doctoral study on preceptorship in nursing conducted in acute and community settings – therefore constitute the major part of this chapter, so that readers can judge for themselves where the findings regarding the development of preceptorship policy and practice in this study have particular relevance for them. Equally well, the findings may be very different from other as yet unreported studies out there in the field.

The claims made for the study described here are that it has:

- Helped to illuminate and clarify some of the problems encountered by practitioners in the implementation of preceptorship policy in the workplace
- Exemplified how preceptorship can be devised and maintained as an organisational strategy for assisting the new in post to adapt to their assumed roles and responsibilities
- Provided a graphic account of the feelings and socialisation processes experienced and shared by staff who collaborated in the study, and an insight into the potential conflicts experienced by staff undertaking the role of preceptor
- Demonstrated the effectiveness of preceptorship in helping the new practitioner to adapt, while at the same time raising some legitimate and widely felt concerns about the use of preceptorship models to support learning at critical stages of career transition
- Clarified some issues regarding professional and institutional policies for managing recruitment, retention and employee development
- Highlighted areas of concern requiring further applied research and policy debate in relation to professional support concepts.

It is not possible to detail here all the activities undertaken as part of the lengthy research process. The reader is referred to the original thesis for such detail, and to a forthcoming text which discusses the problems and attempted solutions experienced by the researcher in arriving at a valid and reliable account of an action research study in professional practice (Morton-Cooper, 1998, 2000 in press).

Issues and concerns raised by the study are applicable across the broad policy area of professional learning support and are in no way confined to nursing, or restricted to the settings in which the research was conducted.

The outcomes of the study and the problems it so graphically relates may also be symptomatic of support systems in other countries and fields of practice, and we look forward to sharing with colleagues further consideration and exploration of policy for future research and development.

Preceptorship in nursing via action research

Background to the study

Until the late 1990s, the means and processes by which new nurses acquire the ability to carry out their practice knowledgeably and with competence remained largely unstudied. Fleck and Fyffe have noted, for example, that there is a strong tendency in evaluative studies of nursing education to focus on learner satisfaction and knowledge acquisition alone, rather than any posited relationship between the quality of learning and the quality of care given to patients and clients consequent to that learning (Fleck & Fyffe, 1997). Previous studies have also tended to examine the techniques and values adopted by learners through their initial education. Whilst worthwhile as an activity in itself, this fails to acknowledge what has become evident in a far-reaching study on the acquisition of nursing roles – that learning about the staff nurse role really begins *after* rather than before qualification (Maben & Macleod Clark, 1997a,b).

In an effort to provide new nurses with structured and appropriate guidance as to what is expected of the qualified nurse here in the researcher's own domicile of the UK, the lead statutory body recommended the introduction of a formal support framework in 1993, one aspect of which concerned the implementation of a learning support partnership known as *preceptorship*. This required employers to prepare and establish preceptorships across the workplace with the stated intent of helping newly qualified practitioners to consolidate existing skills and theoretical knowledge and to develop their practice and interpersonal skills within a supportive and constructive learning environment.

Each newly qualified member of staff (known as the *preceptee*) was to be supported for an agreed period of time (usually four months) by an experienced nurse, midwife or health visitor colleague who had received specific instruction and preparation in the formal role of supporter, hereafter to be described as the *preceptor* (UKCC, 1993). To date, however, no substantive large scale research studies have been made available as to the efficacy or outcomes of preceptorship for education or clinical practice in the UK. Difficulties concerning the definition and transferability of existing preceptor support models, and in particular their practical implementation, have meant that the concept – and practitioners attempting to get to grips with it – have suffered, due in part to the continuing conceptual muddle as to what preceptorship means, but also as a result of the lack of consensus over the relevance and appropriateness of preceptorship practice in different care settings and career situations.

Preceptorship as a means for helping new staff to adjust to and develop their roles as beginning practitioners still constitutes relatively uncharted territory for educationalists and staff developers here in the UK. It was clear from an earlier review of the literature that approaches taken by clinical educators towards beginning practice in nursing in Britain appeared to be extremely variable, and not informed by any extensive critique of the interpersonal or emotional aspects of learning as experienced by staff in the early stages of their careers (Morton-Cooper, 1992). The British nursing establishment could only look on in envy at the apparent ease with which the US and Australian health care systems had appeared to subsume professional learning support into their professional repertoires.

Overall, however, scant attention seems to have been paid to describing the methodology by which experienced nurse preceptors are monitored in the workplace (Allanach, 1988). As Goldenberg *et al.* have noted, while there is no dearth of information on preceptorship *programmes*, there are fewer reports of preceptor's experiences of teaching and learning in the workplace, and most of these have a tendency to be descriptive or anecdotal (Goldenberg *et al.*, 1997, p. 303).

It followed, therefore, that the implementation of preceptorship via an action research study proposed by the present author could be a valuable source of evidence-based information to others. Managed well, a research proposal which afforded both the pragmatic implementation of policy with the systematic appraisal of policy outcomes might not only be of interest and benefit to those involved locally, but could also be of relevance to practitioners across a range of health care disciplines, and not least to the author's own field of practice as an educator of adults.

It was clear from the beginning, then, that any definition of the research problem to be investigated would be purely provisional and dependent for its development and direction on those involved in the policy implementation process. The study needed to be collaborative and involve all relevant practitioners and colleagues as part of a cyclical, reflexive and developmental action research process.

Where research requires some form of intervention it is important to assess the relative merits of quantitative versus qualitative approaches. It is also important for the researcher to respect the potential costs of implementing research findings in advance of any proposed innovation. Organisational costs may be high; changes in procedures or structures are always a challenge. In any health care setting the different workers have evolved specific working relationships which some groups or individuals may have a vested interest in maintaining (Norr, 1994, p. 112).

Local issues and constraints affecting the study

In assessing the potential for any proposed study, it is vital to ascertain the likely stakeholders and to clearly identify those whose interests may be compromised, so that the researcher may at least be aware of potential ethical or financial constraints and any obvious political hurdles to be negotiated as part of the research venture. For example, nursing staff who were to be approached for inclusion in the study anecdotally reported the following difficulties in supporting each other through the critical transition from junior to more experienced member of staff:

- A mismatch between managers and staff performance expectations
- Low morale and a degree of employee disaffection and 'wastage'
- Ineffective performance review systems
- Poor relationships and value conflicts concerning 'attitudes' and job performance
- Some insularity and defensiveness within work teams
- Ambivalence and indifference regarding the problems of newly qualified staff
- Communication difficulties
- No apparent baseline or consistent criteria for measuring the performance of new employees
- An apparent lack of meaningful emotional support for all staff at times of crisis or transfer to an unfamiliar work environment
- Symptoms of reality shock articulated by the newly qualified and new in post
- Flooding of the job market by newly qualified and redeployed nursing staff leading to a freeze on recruitment in some areas with consequent anxiety and low morale amongst nursing students and teaching staff.

Staff were also feeling the impact of the introduction of the UK NHS Patients' Charter, (DoH 1991, 1995), which sought greater accountability and quantification of objectives and outcomes for the service, in answer (at least in part) to a significant increase in the number of litigation cases being brought against health care providers. Any proposed methodology therefore needed to be aware of the prevailing political milieu and of the researcher's likely involvement in managing local and cultural change.

In order to understand the socialisation processes operating in the workplace it was necessary to set up, support and maintain a network of preceptors and preceptee partnerships, and to set appropriate boundaries for the critical examination of the nature of the difficulties associated with beginning practice, thus allowing both parties to properly reflect on their responses, actions and reactions to challenges experienced at work.

We began with just three preceptor pairs in the initial pilot study, graduated to 15 pairs at the beginning of the main study, and by the end some 284 practitioners across five different employers and several sites had joined in – a testimony to the enthusiasm of individual staff to participate, but also to the organisational abilities of key staff in each of the workplaces on whom the study eventually made great demands.

Having begun as a small scale in-depth analysis of local issues and constraints, the study evolved into a much larger scale multi-site project which considered a much broader range of problems and practice related themes, all of which required careful and complex management.

Accounts of beginning practice in nursing

A common plea in qualitative research is the apparent need of the researcher to learn the language and rituals of the informants (Hardey, 1994, p. 63) This is particularly true of studies which attempt to 'get beneath the skin' of a phenomenon. Burman has referred to the 'identification and evaluation of guiding themes or discourses which structure dominant forms', which can then act as a form of critique (Burman, 1994, p. 1).

The dominant forms under scrutiny in our study were those assumptions and practices concerning entry to the workplace for the first few months after qualification and registration, the personal and interpersonal processes of *becoming* a qualified and accountable practitioner, and the rituals surrounding career transitions. The first step came in attempting to identify the *relative importance* (i.e. personal and collective significance) attached to the idea of preceptor support by practitioners involved in the study, all of whom were practising nurses working in a broad range of specialisms and clinical settings.

Constructionist analysis may challenge the ontological status of institutionally recognised and sanctioned phenomena, to ask 'What is the basis of the claim that the phenomena exist at all?' (Sarbin & Kitsuse, 1994, p. 11). As a form of critique, therefore, an examination of how practitioners go about 'constructing', 'describing' and 'explaining' the phenomena they experience could be used to assess the significance and value attached to new role learning within the social world under scrutiny, and to interpret the so-called 'mapping of meaning' referred to in the introductory chapter of this book when we considered the context of health care organisations and levels of trust existing between colleagues.

The views of service managers and educationalists were sought initially, as were those of recently qualified staff and those who had been practising for some time. Those who had responsibility for taking new staff 'under their wing' were also asked for their views on the possibilities offered by preceptorship. First and foremost, the data which emerged from the *pilot study interviews* showed that the need for such a study was much greater than the primary researcher had perhaps appreciated.

When the study began, the recently introduced preceptorship policy (UKCC, 1993) was generally perceived as 'yet something else' to be concerned about, with some disillusionment expressed about the efficacy of any new support arrangement 'when the old ones hadn't worked'. The part played by 'significant others' in the newly qualified nurse's transition to qualified practice was a dominant theme, and in particular the ability of new staff to be able to identify between good, bad and indifferent role models appeared to be a key factor in harnessing the right support for learning during the transition period.

Pilot study data supported the view that a collaborative approach was necessary. For staff nurses in particular, the 'dominant forms' which represented the structures and influences affecting the transitional learning process were *'becoming accountable'* and *'being held responsible'* for what went on in the care of patients and clients. The perceived difference between pre and post-registration practice lay in 'not being allowed to make a mistake like a student would', 'knowing who to go to for help', 'not wanting to feel or look stupid' or forgetful of something other trained staff might consider important.

Interviewees also felt torn between caring for patients and the need to help and guide students and other professionals in the workplace. The more junior nurses expressed guilt at feeling they did not have enough time to support others, which was ironic in that the study was trying to help such nurses access support for themselves. The sense of obligation toward others was acute, with interviewees expressing gratitude for help they felt they had already received in practice, sometimes from unexpected quarters.

Loyalty to colleagues and the work team appeared to be valued highly, and it was difficult at this stage to deduce how much staff wanted to be seen to be loyal to their newly acquired colleagues, rather than being seen to criticise them by describing any failure on their part in supporting them as recent additions to the health care team.

Key concepts which emerged from the pilot study were adjustment, adaptation, coping, getting on with it, looking out for each other and 'learning the ropes'. The pilot study thus provided the primary researcher with some reassurance that preceptorship was in fact a researchable topic and that discourses about transitional learning support processes were clearly to be found in the workplace. The idea that staff should 'work through something together' rather than simply being observed was strongly welcomed by participants.

Special care had to be taken, however, to see that the study did not itself generate a demand for social support which had not existed previously. Clearly we also did not want to foist unwanted support on to a population which had no apparent need for it. It was therefore important to bear in mind that the model of preceptorship offered to participants (now *co-researchers*, in keeping with the ethos of action research principles) might be rejected by staff. The study therefore had to be clearly evaluative, practitioner-generated and work-oriented if it was to hope to be taken seriously as a force for changing and improving existing practice in the field.

Key features of the preceptorship model employed

Confused and inadequate terminology with regard to support concepts was the first and most overwhelming problem to be overcome in the introduction of preceptorship to the workplace. As no standard UK definitions existed at the time, the primary researcher volunteered working definitions based on the literature and adapted to suit British post rather than pre-registration practice. These definitions were refined several times during the period of data collection and constant comparative analysis.

The critical distinction between the established role of pre-registration mentor and the proposed new role of preceptor here in the UK was drawn by defining mentorship as career socialisation and preceptorship as clinical socialisation.

For the purposes of the study a preceptor was defined as:

> 'a qualified and experienced first level nurse who has agreed to work in partnership with a (newly) registered practitioner colleague in order to assist and support them in the process of learning and adaptation to his or her new role.'

> (Morton-Cooper, 1993)

Preceptorship within the study later expanded to take in the transitional learning support offered to all qualified staff who were new in post (rather than just the newly qualified). A more generic definition of preceptorship thus emerged in the study as that of *transitional learning support*, so that when attempting to define preceptorship we did not have to restrict clinical socialisation to those who had just registered. Staff who had transferred or moved to a new area of practice could then be included within the remit of the study, a pragmatic response which went down well with service managers and helped to create and maintain the ethos of collegiality and teamwork in the workplace.

The working model devised for use in the study was based on having *designated preceptors* working in partnership with preceptee colleagues, while *unit preceptors* undertook to manage a group of preceptor pairs and the data collection that their work generated. The relationship between precepting partners was evaluated (primarily, but not exclusively) on the quality of emotional support between the two parties, and was therefore *process* rather than outcomes based. This was a fairly radical departure from the North American models of preceptorship which tend to use instructional and didactic methods for measuring preceptor/preceptee performance, based on the instructor/student dyad model, rather than the peer relationship proposed by the present study.

Five employers provided the resources and time off for co-researchers to receive the preparation required to act as preceptors. This was offered in the form of two day experiential workshops (also described methodologically as *focus groups*), which sought to uncover the values associated with transitional learning and practice.

Values clarification exercises conducted by the primary researcher using the technique of 'Socratic questioning' enabled co-researchers to address Socrates' famous question, 'Is this the right way to live?' – i.e. was our current way of supporting the newly qualified adequate/helpful/ good enough already, or could it be improved in some way in the best interests of all concerned? Co-researchers attending the workshops addressed these questions first of all by examining their own 'significant others' and their recollections of beginning practice (i.e. which kind of support had been helpful and which had not?). They then went on to plan the preceptor support partnership, drawing on available literature and their collective analysis of the issues relevant to their own clinical areas and learning objectives (see appendix to this chapter for a brief outline of the Socratic method).

Reflection on and in practice lay at the centre of our analysis of all written documentation and this took the form of learning diaries, critical incident analyses, process documentation (such as learning contracts, the mutually agreed setting and attainment of personal learning objectives for both preceptee and preceptor) and support group meetings.

Preceptor pairs met regularly over the four month period of support, usually at a prearranged place and time, to discuss mutual expectations of support, to review the learning contracts entered into as part of the support process, and to reflect on examples of both good and bad practice as experienced in the workplace. Some preceptors preferred to work on the same shifts as their preceptees in order to rehearse certain skills.

This proved to be problematic over time, however, as the vagaries of duty rotas, sickness, holidays and other professional development activities sometimes played havoc with their best laid plans. The benefit of having a single record (i.e. the *preceptorship learning contract*) to which both parties could refer did, however, prove vital as it enabled either party to keep in touch with developments on either side at times outside their regular meetings. These were kept in a confidential file held in safe keeping at a designated place of work.

A method of reporting, collecting and coding the data was devised and communicated to unit preceptors, and this provided the main body of text to be transcribed and analysed. Core themes which appeared and reappeared in the literature involved theories related to job strain, stress management, role learning and the qualities needed to develop a 'safe space' for learning which could be tapped into as necessary by co-researchers at different stages. (Some of the key texts which emerged as the most helpful are included under further reading at the end of this chapter.)

The nature of the 'research bargain' entered into between practitioners and the primary researcher was that in exchange for insights gained into transitional learning support, co-researchers were able to develop and refine a system of peer review which had hitherto not been possible using existing support frameworks. The situation for practitioners was relatively straightforward – they implemented the model and changed and refined it to suit local purposes, while the primary researcher provided a synthesis of the processes and research outcomes generated in the form of an empirical model of preceptorship. (The model has since been devised for use across several employers and as such is continuing in the best tradition of action research by carrying on long after the initial problem-solving began).

Practice narratives relating to career transition

For the primary researcher the real focus of interest lay in the interactions and 'stories' produced by practitioners. Fineman and Gabriel capture perfectly the intricacies of story-telling and their strengths as a means of uncovering new knowledge:

> 'The tales told by new entrants to organisations are revealing. Their experiences of work are fresh and sharp, they will 'see' what older hands no longer notice or care about. An articulate, critical but naïve worker can offer poignant insights on the rights and wrongs of

organisational life – its passions, performances, pretences ... they spotlight significant, if transient, moments in organisational life, presented with passion and authenticity.'

(Fineman & Gabriel, 1996, p. 1)

The therapeutic use of stories has a long and distinguished history and is a potent force for personal transformation. Kedar Nath Dwivedi and Damian Gardner believe that the power of telling a story should not be minimised. We structure our lives around specific meanings so that in order to express ourselves and make sense of our lives, we 'story' our experiences and through this process of 'storying' meaning is derived: 'when spoken stories may attain a significance from the context in which they are told' (Dwivedi & Gardner, 1997, p. 23). It is through the available cultural stock of stories that an individual's own stories will be understood and enacted (MacIntyre, quoted in Dwivedi, 1997, p. 22). Such stories are important and need to be heard, particularly if, as educators, we are attempting to be responsive to the needs and concerns of learners. Stories told by co-researchers in this study centred on their experiences of practice based on the following issues:

- What constitutes a 'career transition'. Is the concept of transition a helpful one?
- Is preceptorship needed and if so, why?
- Who are our 'significant others' at home and in the workplace and what influences might/do they have on our values, beliefs, ideas and attitudes?
- What impact do 'personal transitions' have on our emotional lives?
- How can the interpersonal and emotional facets of learning at work be made more explicit to those involved?
- How are the emotional aspects of such learning managed and dealt with in workplace/learner communities?
- What, if any, cultural values predominate in the workplace, and what implications do these have for transitional and professional learning support practice generally?

Preceptorship and 'vocabularies of emotion'

One of the most striking and surprising things about this study has been the development and assimilation of a vocabulary for dealing with the emotions generated by career transitions such as entry to qualified practice. Although the primary researcher had assumed that a language of emotions existed, she was not prepared for the extent to which co-researchers would respond to the appeal for 'emotional data', and for the catharsis provided by the research for the relatively free and unrestrained expression of emotions generally regarding the experience of nursing work.

Earlier reading of studies and texts related to 'emotional labour' (e.g. Hochschild, 1979, 1983; Smith, 1992) had sensitised us to the possibilities of strong emotion or frustration being 'managed' emotionally in the workplace, but the poignant and at times distressing disclosures which emerged as part of the values clarification work both within the workshops and in preceptorship practice was not anticipated.

Emotions and work entry: the importance of 'significant others'

Co-researchers who volunteered to take on the preceptor role had to meet criteria based on UKCC recommendations (UKCC, 1993), and were usually staff nurses who had been qualified for at least two years and who had declared an interest (or had already completed) a course in teaching and assessing in clinical practice. The closer to qualification they were the more empathetic they were towards the problems and fears of the newly qualified, a finding that might have been expected.

More senior staff felt a greater emotional distance between themselves and the newly qualified and were generally less sensitive to the issues and concerns affecting preceptees. When asked to relate their experiences of beginning practice and their own feelings at the time (in small groups and then to the wider forum) the descriptions were startlingly similar over all cohorts. Examples of feelings associated with the transition appear in Box 3.1.

The counterbalance to these overwhelmingly negative replies came from a small minority who saw the experience of transition as a positive one (Box 3.2).

The overwhelming majority of co-researchers cited guilt as the main feeling induced by nursing work. Staff shortages and high expectations of those staff who were working led to feelings of vulnerability and impending crisis, fear of 'what might be just around the corner' and a perceived need to be 'seen to be in control' of whatever happened in their wards or working environments. Those working in the community were especially vulnerable as they often attended patients and clients alone and felt the burden of needing to respond appropriately to whatever demands were made on them.

Co-researchers who participated in the study came from a very wide range of professional backgrounds. These included staff working across all departments in acute general hospital services, staff from learning

Box 3.1

'felt pressurised' 'threatened' 'uncertain and anxious' 'felt left to get on with it – no positive feedback only negative' 'knew I was doing alright when nobody shouted at me' 'was really scared' 'felt conspicuous and uncomfortable' 'demoralised' 'lacked confidence and assertiveness' 'sick to the stomach – had real abdo. pain and insomnia' 'fear of the unknown' 'scared of initiating things and being in charge' 'felt the lack of experience as a student [and] ended up being told, don't think, just do' 'constant fear that somebody will arrest or die' 'felt there was no light at the end of the tunnel, lack of resources ongoing and no solutions offered to the problems day in and dayout' 'unprepared after days off, handovers often poor leading to a feeling of insecurity and chaos' 'relief at having achieved by ambition to qualify' 'lonely' 'fish out of water' 'relatives' expectations put pressure on you' 'relatives know their rights better than I do – I'm aware they can lose me my job' 'scared to approach senior staff in case they think I'm silly or stupid' 'everyone seemed to know more than me, including the patients!' 'didn't feel appreciated for the work I did' 'never enough time to do everything'

Box 3.2

'liked the status being qualified gave me' 'enjoyed the sense of achievement' 'impressed my friends with my new position' 'felt motivated and enthusiastic' 'happy after the worry of qualifying' 'felt important, I knew I mattered suddenly' 'I felt it was character building' 'nervous and excited at wearing the uniform'

disabilities and residential care units, community (i.e. district nursing, midwifery and health visiting staff, nurses working in general practice and community psychiatry). Staff from mainstream psychiatric settings were not closely involved (although they were consulted as part of the initial pilot study) due to the variable clinical supervision. Local experience of clinical supervision in psychiatry was considerable, and it was felt that the distinctive model of learning support already well established locally was likely to be an important variable which would make direct comparative analysis problematic.

Nurses working in high dependency areas seemed to fare well in relation to significant others because the staff–patient ratio was higher, and because there was generally a more experienced and well qualified person around to approach for help and clarification. Nurses in theatres appeared to be the most exposed to negative and demoralising experiences, however, with one nurse encapsulating the feeling of many:

'Hell's bells and buckets of blood ... the psychology of warfare is what it is. What I want to know is, why are we at war with ourselves?'

The notion of being undermined and belittled by nursing colleagues and 'being left to fend for ourselves' was particularly strong in theatres, with a feeling of competitiveness expressed between teams of staff allocated to different theatres or tasks within the theatre complex. This was not exclusive to theatre staff, however. It also occurred with staff working in accident and emergency (A&E) services, although much seemed to depend on the management style of the person in overall charge, either the A&E manager or the casualty consultant. Where junior doctors were considered to be helpful and considerate the reports were more positive and this held generally across all cohorts and areas of care. Where junior doctors were thought to be equally out of their depth, respondents expressed some sympathy and/or empathy for the doctors' position, but expressed concern and resentment that nurses should be expected to make up the shortfall for the doctor's lack of experience or know-how:

'It's not like we're experienced or anything. They look to us for help and if they don't get it the first time they tend to think we're not up to it and ignore us when we do give advice or make suggestions...'

The quality of the relationship between doctors and nurses seemed to be an important indicator of the overall ethos and atmosphere in the workplace. Although it was expected that the senior consultant or the ward manager would be an important influence on this process, in reality participants expressed strong feelings about those staff who were working closest to them. 'Cliquishness' and 'taking over because they're quicker' were frequently cited when participants were asked to identify what had specifically helped or hindered them. For staff who had taken up appointment in wards or areas where they had previously been allocated as nursing students, the relationships were generally more stable and positive, presumably because they had based their decision to apply for a job on earlier positive experiences. Again, however, this could not be relied on, as staff changeovers and turnover, work re-organisations, variable levels of sickness absence and maternity leave sometimes meant that strategic changes had to be made at short notice.

Newly qualified nurses expecting one scenario were therefore not always guaranteed the colleagues they had anticipated. This seemed to add to the isolation felt by new staff, and was particularly acute where staff were expected to fill in for colleagues working in other areas at short notice. The unfamiliarity of the surroundings and the idiosyncrasies of different routines loomed large for the inexperienced nurse who was attempting to fit into the prevailing system, and lack of time to attend to the details of particular environments seemed to lead to a feeling of disorientation expressed as 'confusion' or 'fish out of water' analogies.

When asked to describe individuals who helped or hindered their transition to the new role, the picture was equally vivid (Box 3.3).

Box 3.3

Hindrances included:
'unapproachable staff' 'grouchy, hard-pressed doctors' 'people opposed to change and suggestions for change from the newly qualified' 'consultants who throw their weight around' 'lack of knowledge about the role' 'being frightened of being accountable' 'scared of the legal consequences, kept checking and cross-checking everything [un]til it drove everybody mad' 'bossy relatives' 'warned not to step out of line' 'trained [experienced and more senior] staff unable to take criticism or open their eyes to new ideas' 'felt theoretically confident but practically useless' 'didn't always feel confident about the consequences of certain actions' 'felt like work was an initiation test' 'felt like I had to prove I wouldn't be disloyal' 'scared to own up to my mistakes unless I heard somebody else do it first' 'paranoid about cliquey staff'

Identification of 'significant others' in the transition process

The task of identifying those individuals who had actively or indirectly supported the transition process was an enlightening task for participants as many were reflecting on the process publicly and privately for the first time. By far the most supportive 'significant others' identified (contrary to the literature on the role played by the traditional ward sister in the past) were the army of unqualified but very experienced staff on the wards such as health care assistants and support workers. The consensus seemed to be that if you gained the confidence of the most experienced support worker then your position was that much more secure. Gain his/her poor opinion of your abilities and your problems would magnify accordingly!

Senior managers did not really figure at all in participants' analyses of significant others, other than negatively. Feelings associated with managers tended to centre on whether resources were managed effectively or ineffectively, or whether more senior staff sidelined the newly qualified nurse, giving other colleagues preference. Provided managers took only a friendly and pastoral interest in the newly qualified (by implication not interfering in the day to day work of the nurses) they could 'just about be tolerated' as a part of the workforce. Should a manager intervene in some way, perhaps by commenting on the performance of the new member of staff, then managers were deemed to have a potentially punitive impact on the individual.

Contact between the very senior and/or experienced staff did not seem to be expected or encouraged: rather, considerable distance between the two appeared to be the preferred strategy as far as the newly and recently qualified were concerned. Conversely, where managers were unable to recognise and acknowledge new members of staff or remember their names, they came in for particularly vitriolic criticism for not being 'in touch' with the grassroots level of the service. This seemed to be something of a contradiction in terms. Managers' interest was effectively discouraged while their apparent disinterest was condemned as a lack of care or concern for the staff 'who were keeping the service going.'

This hinted at a more complex role for nurse managers than has perhaps been appreciated or evident in the literature, and seemed to suggest that the transition from service to business manager within the consumer ethos of the NHS has had more subtle effects on the culture than had previously been realised.

Other helpers in the transition process included friends, neighbours, family and colleagues working within the new nurse's own team. Personality clashes between colleagues did not seem to be a huge problem, although where these were expressed the impact seemed to have fairly devastating consequences for the individuals concerned.

It soon became clear that opportunities to resolve these personality conflicts would be an important aspect of any learning support role. Given changes in clinical leadership and the development of flatter organisational hierarchies within the health care system, not all problems depended on the actions, opinions or responses of the most senior member of staff. The legendary power of the traditional ward sister/charge nurse appears to have dissipated somewhat in this regard, with nurses expecting to have more say in the decision-making processes associated with the management of care.

Significant others who were singled out for particular praise were those experienced enrolled nurses who had not yet converted to first level practice. Their fund of knowledge and practical experience of ward routines, familiarity with procedures and established position within the health care team meant that they were in a solid position to offer support to the newly qualified. Unlike their staff nurse colleagues they appeared to feel less threatened by the presence of the newly qualified, perhaps perceiving the new nurses' worries about being able to deliver care effectively in the light of educational reforms and their perceived inferior practical experience in relation to their newly acquired acquired theoretical knowledge base. Enrolled nurses seemed to be particularly skilled at appearing at the new nurse's shoulder just as an 'experienced hand' was needed.

The knock-on effect of this was sometimes negative, however, as it had a tendency to make the newly qualified feel even more inadequate, by appearing to confirm cultural prejudices and beliefs that the new system of nurse education in higher education institutions was 'not working and not all that it's cracked up to be'. In this sense those newly qualified in the last ten years have been put into the unenviable position of having to defend their formal standards of pre-registration preparation (i.e. Project 2000) as well as their own performance in relation to earlier traditional methods of training. Examples of this competitive attitude emerging between traditionally trained and diplomate nurses included: 'If you suggested something different then it was a third world war', 'she came to us qualified never having taken a blood pressure', 'she told me she hadn't come into nursing to deal with patients but to lead from the front. What kind of nurse is that can you tell me?'

The most positive comments came from staff who had decided to call a truce over this particular argument and those who 'saved face' by recognising the contribution to be made from both traditionally and recently qualified staff, arguing that what one lacked the other could rectify in the best interests and practices brought about by team working. One ward even incorporated this ethos into its published philosophy of care by claiming to uphold a 'shared learning ethos' between staff across the multi-disciplinary team.

Other factors affecting transition

Regarding other factors which were thought to help the transition process, several other critical strategies emerged. When asked to put forward their own successful strategies for dealing with new role learning, some offerings were decidedly tongue-in-cheek: 'Benson & Hedges and Holsten Pils!', 'fags, snooker and long nights out'. It was interesting to pick up the gender issues here, in that the men in the cohorts (a minority of some 26, $n = 284$) were much less comfortable about discussing their experiences or feelings openly.

With the notable exception of critical incident analysis, which all participants took very seriously, the men seemed to be more comfortable with a lighter, more humorous approach to disclosure. Some groups were markedly more sensitive to these nuances of feeling than others. For example, where more than one man was included in the group the discussions rarely veered into the expression of acute feelings of sadness or bewilderment. Frustrations tended to be framed in the language of conflict with the frequent expression of anger, disgust or even betrayal from the men, in distinct contrast to the guilt-edged responses of female participants. For the men, the problems were attributed to a faulty and uncaring system; for the women, it was more a question of feeling guilty for their own inadequacies in coming to terms with their new roles.

Role-making and *role-taking* are influenced by the specific ideas people have about 'proper, normal, and expectable [sic] conduct for boys or girls, men or women' (Hewitt, 1994, p. 127), and presumably (in this case) by those enacting and participating in this thing we call 'nursing'. The shift from traditional notions of selfless giving required of nurses in the formative Nightingale era of the 1860s, to the development of what has recently been described as the 'new nursing', has involved a redefining of the meaning and boundaries of the nursing role, so that:

> 'the meaning of nursing care appears to be shifting from the requirement of nurses to understand and address the patient's needs (caring for), towards a broader interpretation which includes both 'caring for' and 'caring about' [patients] ...'

> (Savage, 1995, p. 51)

This implies a much stronger political emphasis on the role of the nurse as patient's advocate, so that the apparent aggression expressed by the men in the present study need not necessarily be 'male' at all, but rather constitute new evidence to illustrate the culture shift nursing is experiencing in its drive for professional autonomy and status. It should also be mentioned, however, that men in the present study saw themselves (in the main) as 'bi-cultural troublemakers' (after Kramer, 1974), charged with the task of 'bringing nursing into the twenty-first century', and of assimilating the qualities and attributes of the 'new nurse' with the more openly competitive and market-oriented system of health care being offered. They appeared to share the same high aspirations and commitment to patient care as their female colleagues. The difference seemed to lie with different conceptions of 'service', hence rather than adhering to notions of servility and humility – a position favoured by the nineteenth century traditionalist ethos – they preferred to conceptualise nursing as a 'service' in much the same vein as other services within the more contemporary idea of 'service sector employment'.

This also highlighted the potential conflict experienced by different staff attributing different cultural values to the idea of providing and maintaining different aspects of service. For some, nursing was about supervising and directing care holistically and with regard to ethical principles; for others, it was about maintaining a good nurse–patient relationship.

This was the first of several areas of conflict to emerge in the study between co-researchers, and it marked the beginning of the important exploration and clarification of values which was to constitute the next stage of the investigation.

The next matter for consideration concerned the identification, availability and trustworthiness of significant others to assist with transition in the workplace.

Confronting the question: Who is most suited to the preceptor role?

Having identified the likely candidates to enact the preceptor role (i.e. support workers and enrolled nurses), an insoluble problem emerged. Policymakers had already decreed that only experienced first level nurses could act as preceptors. On balance, the evidence acquired to date suggested that they were in fact possibly the worst candidates for the role!

How were the action researchers in the present study to address this problem and arrive at a satisfactory solution for all concerned? It was now becoming clear to the staff nurses acting as co-researchers that *they were themselves the problem* confronting the newly qualified. Having assessed and found their staff nurse and more senior colleagues wanting in the business of providing transitional support, they now had the thorny problem of raising awareness and changing attitudes within their own ranks. The convenient distinction between 'them' and 'us' was disappearing fast. How did they feel about this insight, and how enlightened did they expect other colleagues to become in the light of this new-found knowledge?

Even when asked to identify factors which enhanced the transition or which 'made life easier', co-researchers had a good deal of trouble in articulating what these people or strategies might be. Again, emphasis was firmly on the negative. Responses ranged from 'always one member of staff who is unapproachable and unkind', 'abrupt relatives can make your life miserable', to the (slightly!) more encouraging 'filling me in on the ward gossip was a help – I knew who to avoid, then', or 'demands changed with putting on the staff nurses' uniform; the doctors didn't expect any different [from you], you might have been qualified for five years or five minutes, it was all the same to them'.

The night staff came in for particularly bitter criticism:

'No-one said what happened on nights, so when I went on for the first time I was late doing the drugs [round]. Night sister came on demanding to know why I was still doing the drugs at 11.30 [p.m.]. I burst into tears – I felt I'd been up to something I shouldn't be doing. I avoided her in the future, she was so nasty.'

Hopes pinned on support from other staff sometimes had unexpected consequences:

'It was better to get on and do it, rather than thinking about it. I had the problem moving from kids [paediatrics] to the medical unit. The change was horrendous, nobody helped but the auxiliaries. I was allocated a mentor – another member of staff – but after the fourth shift on that fell apart. The sister was very good giving me an idea about what she expected and the [ward] procedures and so on, but it was the EN [enrolled nurse] who took me under her wing. Told me the gossip and who not to rub up the wrong way...'

'The ward sister everybody'd warned me about sat me down and said that I wasn't to take everything to myself. She said that if things didn't go quite right then everybody had a share in putting it right. She wanted to be the first, not the last to know. That was sort of reassuring for me, knowing that somebody was looking out for me and wouldn't be surprised if it didn't fall into place right away.'

Discussions concerning the rights and wrongs of practice and the example set by more experienced staff tended to focus on the identification of an empathetic person who would 'be there' for the new nurse. The skills required by the beginning practitioner therefore included the ability to differentiate between a 'good' role model and one who would be 'a bad influence', or have a negative effect on their self-confidence.

However, when asked how new nurses could be expected to tell the difference between good and bad role models, co-researchers had some difficulty in formulating a strategy for their preceptees. To begin with, they put into words what they saw to be the attributes of a positive role model:

- Approachability – accessibility
- Calm and in control – sense of humour
- Kind to patients – has high standards [of care]
- A safe practitioner – up to date

- Well motivated – can be trusted with personal and or confidential information
- Understanding – has empathy
- Adaptable – has a friendly personality
- Smart appearance – is assertive
- A good communicator – has good leadership skills
- Somebody you would like to be like
- Someone who can justify their actions
- Knowledgeable and clinically skilled
- Keeps a professional distance – is firm but fair
- Inspires confidence – is truthful, commands respect, has organisational ability.

Other qualities described concerned the ability to admit or 'own up to mistakes', to be someone 'who follows guidelines', who is 'research-minded', who 'sets a good example', someone 'who can prioritise efficiently' and 'pull their weight'.

By contrast, poor role models were:

- Those who 'broke the rules' – 'bad listeners', 'dressed sloppily'
- 'Saw patients as a burden' – 'those who were quick to criticise'
- Those with an abrupt or 'superior' manner
- Those who 'badmouthed' the system or each other.

Enabling/disabling strategies

Palmer would view these different characteristics as *enabling* and *disabling*. The most effective supporters in her view would be those who are open and constructive, and who enable by being accessible, responsive to the needs of others, easy to trust, being comfortable with themselves and their abilities, and by being able to command mutual respect. Disablers, in contrast, are inaccessible, throw people into new roles using 'sink or swim' strategies, refuse requests, over-supervise, and destroy by 'dumping' on another person or by openly criticising them in front of their colleagues. In addition, however, there are the all important and influential 'enabling disablers' or 'enabling manipulators' who appear to be helpful superficially, but whose actions of creating tensions and disruption exert a much more subtle, but equally devastating, effect as rank disablers on individuals by *seeming* to provide support when in fact the reverse is true.

This categorisation of enabling–disabling traits was a very helpful one for the present study, in that it allowed co-researchers to frame helpful strategies from a non-manipulative, facilitative point of reference, building on the positive attributes while taking into account the need for supporters to appear human in the eyes of anxious neophytes (see pages 49–51 of the first edition for a discussion on these issues).

Clarification of the differences between good and bad role models could be acquired through sensitivity to enabling/disabling traits, so that the overriding issue for the staff nurse or colleague trying to provide support was, 'Is this an enabling or disabling thing to do?' This had obvious implications for staff who liked to dominate or bully less experienced staff, or who added to their uncertainties by undermining their new-found authority as a qualified member of staff.

Feelings management and the issue of control

Another of the themes which recurred throughout the study was that of 'feelings management', of coping with the emotional onslaught brought on by caring for others, and for maintaining some sort of emotional equilibrium in the face of constant demands for attention. In examining the connections between role enactment and moral sensitivity, Scott (1995, p. 328) comments that health care practitioners should recognise that 'in taking on the role of nurse or doctor she/he is taking on a par-ticular role with identifiable rights and duties'. Scott contends that the relationship between role enactment and moral strategy should be sta-ted more explicitly than it is at present, so that new practitioners have a more realistic expectation of the role intended for them.

Patients' well-being depends on the skill with which practitioners are able to empathise and care for them. Understanding and sensitivity to the patient's uniqueness are critical to the success of care delivery:

> 'For those working in areas such as caring for the old or long-term sick people it soon becomes apparent ... that the way in which medical and nursing staff relate to and interact with these patients can mean the difference between patients retaining a sense of reality and a normally functioning personality or feeling forced to revert to childish manipulation or the throwing of temper tantrums in order to gain some sense of control over their environment.'
>
> (Scott, 1995, p. 326)

The need to stay in control of this work environment, to be able to respond adequately to the daily round of physical and emotional demands pressed on them was, as had been hinted at in the literature review, an over-arching theme of the nursing discourse engendered by this study. At the heart of this lay fear: fear of failure, 'fear of letting the side down', fear of failing colleagues and patients in the necessary life-saving or life-enhancing activities which made up the work of nurses. Above all, lay the spectre of accountability, a fear of the responsibilities surrounding *accountable practice.*

Accountability and the issue of 'standards'

The nurses within this study set themselves extremely high standards and then seemed prepared to punish themselves and their colleagues if such standards were not maintained. Accountability, it was concluded, meant 'being able to justify your actions', 'being answerable to others for your actions', 'taking the rap for what goes wrong'.

In attempting to raise standards within nursing, the statutory bodies, which were created in 1983 following on from the 1979 Nurses, Midwives and Health Visitors' Act, would therefore appear to have succeeded in their drive to make nurses respectful of their many responsibilities and duties. In a recent textbook on accountability aimed at nurses Chalmers states:

> 'Accountability thrives in professional groups with a sound know-ledge base, with a high level of skill, with a clear commitment to improving standards and with the maturity and confidence to tackle difficult decisions knowing that there will be management and professional support. Accountability flounders where there is inadequate knowledge, underdeveloped skills, little motivation, a lack of self-confidence and a fear of reprisals. The exercising of accountability is an indication of a professional group that has reached a certain maturity and values accountability as a necessary means of building on that maturity.'

> (Chalmers, 1995, p. 36)

The feelings and situations described in this study would therefore appear to reflect two things. On the face of it, a lack of professional and managerial support is to blame for not allowing nurses to achieve their aims. An examination of the policy and management literature, however, shows that managers and more senior practitioners grapple with the same problems as their more junior colleagues: ill-defined roles, a mismatch of expectations, constant shifts in policy, and feelings of exasperation at not appearing to meet the demands made on them.

An over-weening emphasis on managerial effectiveness and performance management has led managers to search for ways to increase 'situational sensitivity', so that 'the manager is helped to develop the

capacity to interpret his or her situation accurately so that they understand fully what is expected of them, and is then helped to enhance or
develop the skills and capabilities that will allow them to meet those
expectations.' (Flanagan & Spurgeon, 1996, p. 20)

The problem with this approach is that it assumes that some sort of
natural order is both possible and achievable, even under difficult and
challenging conditions. The evidence for nurses involved in this study,
refutes this assumption absolutely. As Brykczynska (1993) has com-
mented:

> 'When value systems conflict between an individual and the col-
> lective or the institution or profession, then *inter-personal moral
> distress* may develop' [italics added].

> (Brykczynska, 1993, p. 137)

Thus the demand for order in the face of massive structural disorder
places a heavy burden on health care practitioners, particularly when
it is realised that they are expected to serve many different 'masters',
i.e. patients and their loved ones, managers, colleagues, the professional ideal, their own professional self-image and concept, their families, friends and 'society' generally, in the UKCC's standard
exhortation that:

> 'Each registered nurse, midwife or health visitor, shall act, at all
> times, in such a manner as to: safeguard and promote the interests
> of individual patients and clients; serve the interests of society;
> justify public trust and confidence and uphold and enhance the
> good standing and reputation of the professions.'

> (UKCC, 1996, p. 8)

On reading the UKCC's document on accountability, it is easy to see why
nurses are doomed to failure. Selflessness is still required of them as the
21st century approaches, to the point of 'making sure that you put the
interests of patients, clients and the public before your own interests and
those of your professional colleagues' (UKCC, 1996, p. 9).

The UKCC's amended Guidelines for Professional Practice (1996) go
on to pile yet more pressure on practitioners by clarifying their
responsibilities for making managers aware of shortcomings in the
work environment. Yet where nurses have effectively 'blown the whis-
tle' to attract attention to poor practice or working conditions, 'the
system' has been largely unsympathetic to their cries for help, with
attempts to 'scapegoat' and demean the individual, so that 'raising jus-

tified grievances may ... put their posts in jeopardy' (Dimond, 1994, p. 70).

Dimond warns that staff who whistleblow cannot necessarily look to their colleagues for support, as strike action or any industrial work-to-rule is not ethically acceptable to many practitioners and is probably in breach of the UKCC Code of Professional Conduct anyway:

> 'There are no signs that the UKCC is able or prepared to take public action for those practitioners who find themselves in a Catch 22 dilemma. This is a serious situation and one which should be considered by the Government and the statutory bodies in order to ensure that standards are maintained.'

> (Dimond, 1994, p. 70)

If accountability has therefore not been welcomed by nurses, as Chalmers decrees (Chalmers, 1995, p. 37), it is no wonder and no surprise as to why.

There is precious little escape for nurses under the present system, so that venting of emotions is an unwelcome adjunct to the pressure of the 'put up and shut up' philosophy which constitutes the hidden curriculum in nursing work. As the economist Catherine Casey has maintained, this may be evidence of the change from industrial to post-industrial forms of work. She argues that the primary impact of work is no longer on the body – the need for physical prowess demanded by bodily exertion and created bodily fatigue – but rather the post-industrial requirement for capturing 'the quick, attentive, trained mind', for example, in the corporate identity. Even at the low-paid, lower-skilled end of the service sector where the stamina to do physical work is needed, additional skills of 'personality', 'congeniality', good humour and interactive skills are required:

> 'The discursive or communicational practices of work not only socialise "normal" adaptive workers into work tasks and habits, they fundamentally affect one's emotional and psychic processes, sense of well-being and identity.'

> (Casey, 1995, p. 86)

Taking this a pragmatic stage further, nurses not only have to put their hands and heart into their work, but their souls are required as well.

The development of 'stressometers'

When asked to name the aspects of the role which caused them concern, nurses within the present study constructed various models of analysis, including an illuminating and easy to use 'stressometer'. Drawn figuratively as a fairground hammer and bell, nurses were asked to name stressors or challenging situations and to 'rate' them according to their perceived level of emotional pressure. The top of the bell constituted a maximum score of 100, whilst the least pressure on the hammer constituted the zero score.

Taking all of the stressometers into account, difficulties or positive challenges encountered did not correlate with what were consensually perceived to be the worst stressors. For example, caring for the dying or resuscitation of a very sick patient were agreed to be the most feared aspects of nursing work. Making a drug administration error came a close third.

In theory, therefore, these aspects of care could be expected to be the most stressful and emotionally laden. But when asked to rate different stressors these actually came quite low on the scale, perhaps because they were not everyday occurrences. Dealing with death and bereavement therefore achieved an average score of 40, while everyday headaches, such as dealing with routine paperwork or managing the doctors' ward round, accumulated a much heavier score of 80 and were rated as a constant stressor over an occasional one.

The conclusion reached by participants was that the major stressors were not in fact major after all, as the perceived 'minor' stressors had a much more damaging cumulative effect on the mental workload of practitioners. Contrary to the primary researcher's expectations, there was in no sense any conceptualisation of an emotional 'reserve' for dealing with stressful events. Rather, each day seemed to be perceived as a 'new' day. The thought of mentally piling up different stressors and then counting their effects was considered too dangerous or demoralising for participants. This 'one day at a time' philosophy seemed to be integral to any sense of personal order, control and/or stability for individuals.

Some preceptors in the study were so taken with the notion of a 'barometer of emotional health' that personal 'stressometers' were encouraged as part of the learning support process, with preceptees being asked to define and reflect on their personal stressors as they experienced them in day to day activities. Their use seemed to offer a means of helping to establish some level of emotional control over the high demands made on new practitioners, and also gave experienced nurses an insight into those areas of care or management which might usefully be managed better. An important benefit which seemed to have been derived from the study was the opportunity that preparing for preceptorship gave to trained staff to reflect on their own capabilities and practice. This was not all plain-sailing, however, as the discussion which follows will demonstrate.

The support paradox

Related to this problem of identifying stressors was the paradox created by preceptor support. This was the finding that those who proved to be the most approachable and expert at providing support carried a much heavier emotional load than their less accessible colleagues. Certain individuals were able to establish a better rapport with newcomers, appeared to be more sympathetic to their fears and aspirations, and were better able to convey this understanding in a way which attracted individuals to them and captured their attention.

In the main, such people were also ready to volunteer themselves and become more emotionally involved with prospective preceptees, so that when the time came for ward managers to allocate a preceptor, certain names fell more easily into the proverbial hat. This was a problem for everyone, because not only did this place an unfair burden on the individual concerned, it also allowed others within the team to delegate and absent responsibility for providing support in the hope that this person would leave them 'to get on with other things'.

The effect of this was to polarise responsibility for support exclusively into the preceptor camp. This was especially hard for some preceptors, particularly where they were also assessors of practice and therefore had responsibility for assessing the work of students as well as the trained staff. Whilst some preceptors initially thrived on 'the need to be needed', others soon found that other aspects of their work suffered, to the detriment of their own personal development and, occasionally (it was perceived), their prospects for promotion. This latter charge, however, has over time been proved to be unfounded, in that a substantial number of preceptors in the present study acquired quicker than usual promotion to higher grades or other jobs, the reasons for which are open to some speculation.

Unit preceptors have argued that preceptors grew in confidence and acquired the respect of other colleagues for being able to carry out their own roles on top of the demands made on them as a preceptor/researcher. Others have maintained that only the 'high-fliers' in an organisation would ever volunteer for preceptorship anyway, thus seeing and capitalising on the opportunity it provides for proving one's mettle.

The primary researcher suspects the answer may lie somewhere between these two arguments, with some preceptors anticipating a career move, while others were genuinely able to reflect and make career decisions for themselves by virtue of the self-scrutiny offered to them by involvement in the study. Evidence for this exists in the small number who decided that nursing was not, after all, the career for them. The preceptor role was also the catalyst for other life decisions, such as coming to terms with their own sexuality, starting a family or changing specialisms within nursing.

Overall, the interpersonal learning process offered participants the chance to examine their personal beliefs and priorities very carefully. Given the unreliability of exit interviews for establishing the real cause as to why employees leave the organisation, it is virtually impossible to establish which actions were the direct result of involvement in preceptorship, and those which might have occurred naturally anyway.

The support paradox is, however, something which was firmly established in the minds of co-researchers, and as such it should inform future policy decisions.

The politics of skill rehearsal: preceptors as judge and jury

Interviews with preceptor pairs and with individuals highlighted issues of peer support affecting the implementation of formal support in the workplace. From a nursing perspective, it was found that the relationship fared much better when formal assessment of performance was effectively removed from the support process. By keeping strictly to a supportive non-judgemental ethos, both parties found it much easier to admit to feelings of inadequacy, to share misgivings and fears, and to disclose important personal information which might have been considered prohibitive under conditions requiring a formal judgement of preceptee performance.

This decision was, however, a major departure from previous models of preceptorship, where some considered analysis of the preceptee's ability to meet set objectives to be closer to the norm. It was found that the problem with performance assessment is that it denies the partners in the relationship a feeling of true reciprocity.

One health employer who did not take part in this study informed the researcher that the purpose of the preceptorship support period of four months was to identify those who were competent from those who were not. Accordingly, the practice of that employer was to set particular behavioural and task objectives for the new appointee, on the basis that should they fail to meet requirements by the end of the four month 'support' period, their contracts would not be renewed.

At a meeting with UKCC representatives in 1992 the present researcher had also been told categorically that preceptorship was not intended as a probationary period for the newly qualified, as this would suggest some concern with Project 2000 nurses being perceived as unable to meet the competencies required for qualified practice. Thus, even though the statutory body responsible for professional standards was clear in this regard, this did not prevent employers from interpreting their intentions differently. Any suggestion that contracts of employment should be hidebound by preceptorship was therefore anathema to some participants, who saw 'top–down' objectives as a potential 'stick to beat new nurses with', as a coercive and restrictive practice which would severely limit the autonomy of nurses, and which would make any hope of a mutually satisfactory relationship between preceptor and preceptee unlikely.

From the employer's point of view, however, it could be argued that this seemed to be a rational if 'knee-jerk' response to concerns being expressed over the practical competence of P2000 diplomate staff. Even more interesting for co-researchers in the present study was the development of a system of peer review through preceptorship, as not only did preceptors have the opportunity to 'shadow', guide and comment on the difficulties encountered by their preceptees, but they too found their practice under scrutiny by themselves and by their more junior colleagues. In the interviews with preceptor pairs it was clear that this gave both partners the valuable opportunity to enter into and examine the rationales for each other's actions and responses to situations, and to gain insight into different ways of meeting the demands made on them.

In the present study both partners were surprised to acknowledge the provisional nature of many decisions made about practice. While mistakes or errors made by the preceptee could be dealt with using policy guidelines, a much more intractable problem emerged when the more experienced preceptor showed weaknesses or errors of judgement in day-to-day practice. No-one who was present at the beginning stages of this study had considered the possibility that the preceptors would be anything other than exemplary in their conduct or actions; so that, while early provision was made for the eventuality of any preceptee error, no guidelines were in place for dealing with preceptors who fell below the standards expected of them.

The problems encountered by preceptor pairs were brought more fully to light when one-to-one interviews were conducted, and when personal disclosures were made by individuals as to the ways in which either party felt let down by the other. One preceptee, for example, felt that:

"The cosy relationship we had was OK until she dropped this terrible clanger and told the wrong person their relative had died. I was on the same shift and she [the preceptor] came over to me and started to cry and asked me what she should do now ... I was taken aback ... Here was this person I'm supposed to look up to and she's all over the place and dropping clangers like that ... It made me wonder what my chances were when somebody that experienced could still get it wrong.'

Preceptors felt the need to set a good example:

'We're very like chalk and cheese. Sometimes I felt like the big, bad ogre always on his back for this or that. At one stage I was getting extremely upset at him for not pulling his weight. I was shouting and saying that OK, if he wanted to sink he could sink, but he wasn't going to do it on my ward. He'd been difficult and stroppy as a student and nobody's tackled this problem head on. The school [of nursing] were aware of it and so were the senior staff, here; now it was left up to me to sort him out. When his timekeeping got really bad I withdrew my approval and he didn't like that. Then I felt bad – thinking who am I to boss him about like this? Still – he had to learn or he'd sink, wouldn't he?'

On the rare occasions where preceptors made an important error which threatened to have serious consequences for a patient, the issue of whether that person should continue as a preceptor was lost amidst procedural matters designed to protect the patient. Where preceptees actually witnessed the error, or challenged a preceptor's decision over care, real anguish was experienced at times over whether to try and gloss over difficulties, or whether to deal with the situation together. Ultimately, relationships either survived or perished, depending on the outcomes of the situation and the level of mutual emotional and psychological support felt in the relationship. Where mutual trust was broken (for example, when a preceptor lied to a manager that he had been consulted by a preceptee before an action was taken), the relationship broke down completely and considerable difficulties were experienced by unit preceptors/co-ordinators in picking up the pieces of the relationship and dealing with the procedural aftermath. One preceptee caught the message accurately here when she said that:

'... honesty is important in the preceptor relationship. Honesty can be hard sometimes, but you don't just want the preceptor to be nicey–nicey supportive or you won't learn from your mistakes...'

Perceived benefits to patients

A major benefit for patients of the preceptor support network was that of finding 'two heads better than one' in resolving day-to-day problems in the workplace. Where previously a lone practitioner might have highlighted a problem, too little power or influence might lead to a failure to take restorative action. With the support of an experienced practitioner behind them, even inexperienced beginners had an advocate.

This led to substantial changes in practice in some working environments, not least in the conditions and practices affecting the lifting, handling and pre/post-operative care of patients, patient communication, dealing with bereavements and the more humane transfer of patients from one department to another. The use of critical incident analysis to highlight particularly good or bad examples of practice helped preceptor pairs to make provisional plans for possible future courses of action and encouraged them to make up the perceived gaps in their knowledge base, and to influence policy and practice at a tangible and influential level.

It was increasingly clear from discussions conducted in preceptor support meetings, however, that the successful conduct of preceptorship depended heavily on the 'troubleshooting' skills of the unit preceptor. Designated ward (or area) preceptors felt that they would be lost without being able to call on the unit preceptor for help and information on hospital or community policies. This may, in part, have been because unit preceptors were high profile, experienced and much respected nurses in the organisation, and as such it was natural that less experienced nurses should turn to them for guidance when they encountered problems in the workplace.

What has not, and cannot yet, be evaluated, is the extent to which unit preceptors were responsible for the relative smooth-running of the preceptorship network, as to grasp some measure of their influence a comparative study leaving out the unit preceptor contribution would have to be carried out.

The costs of caring: does preceptorship help to reduce these?

Preceptorship in nursing has already been declared an 'inadequate and ambiguous response to the quality of pre-registration education, the role of the nurse tutor, the inadequacy of clinical teaching and rostered service, and the validity and utility of nursing theory' (Bowles, 1995, pp. 25–8). Bowles argues that the principal effects of formal preceptorship are to shift the burden of responsibility and accountability from educationalists onto clinical staff and the organisations which employ them; this may effectively divert much needed resources from patient care, and contribute to 'a decline in educational standards, in particular with regard to the practical clinical skills among newly registered nurses' (Bowles, 1995).

The findings of this study would certainly concur with Bowles' assertion that too high a burden is being placed on clinical staff, and that the recent review commissioned by the statutory bodies was right to re-examine its understanding of competence, and reconsider the standards to be achieved by the newly qualified (UKCC, 1999). Unrealistic expectations on the part of staff at all grades and in a variety of speci-alisms may have much to do with the culture of negativity currently affecting qualified nurses, so that some considered reappraisal of the costs and benefits of challenging the ideal in nursing needs to be urgently realised. As Farmer has written:

> 'We can all remember times of suffering in our professional lives. Sometimes the hurt is of a personal nature; more often we suffer because we have failed to respond to the needs of our patients and clients. Rationalising about associated factors such as scarcity of resources as a reason for our impotence seldom alters the sense of failure, or relieves the pain that is its product. Failure to act on behalf of patients or to support colleagues in a fight for justice is a failure to care, and to exercise the power that is inherent in caring.'

(Farmer, 1993, p. 33)

The difficulty is that such an appeal to nurses not to abuse their power in caring for people places yet more onus on individuals to fight social injustice, and to reckon with the 'forces of darkness' which appear to undermine their advocacy of the vulnerable public. It is perhaps no coincidence that nurses lead the way for women who commit suicide. More than 5% of all suicides in the 10 years to 1992 were nurses; some 523 nurses are said to have killed themselves (Mullin, 1996, p. 3).

In the pursuit of 'the right way to live' therefore it is important to maintain some sense of emotional balance when considering the pres-sures on individuals, so that the vagaries of the system do not become the sole responsibility of those charged with caring. The 'reductionist' approach to health care, typified by market principles, must force nur-ses, in Ellis' view, to ask, 'what cost caring?' (Ellis, 1992).

However, it is evident from the data trawled for this study, and from the concepts and constructs which informed it, that the meanings inferred and the problems faced are much greater than any simple value conflict with prevailing power structures in meeting health care demand.

Rather, they force a critical examination of nurses' own expectations of their conduct, and of the need to develop greater emotional literacy, so that instead of turning inwards to punish themselves, nurses might connect with the wider world, to see that elsewhere people are experiencing a similarly 'damaged life' in the postmodern sense (Sloan, 1996).

By recognising the wider social influences at work nurses may thus be relieved of this sense of burden, of paralysing fear of failure, with the possibility for then exploring and challenging the cultural assumptions which expect them to put their own emotional and physical needs last. Nurses are not the angels the popular media would profess them to be. They are human, and should be able to say so from a position of influence in the caring work that they do. Nurses will often feel bruised and confused when they enter the arena of public policy debate (Davies, 1995, p. 187), but that is no reason to withdraw from the arena. A revitalisation of public life and a rethinking of the key institutions of social welfare are within their grasp and, if Davies is right, they may be able to help us move on from the 'limited visions of reform' here in the UK which characterised health care in earlier years (Davies, 1995, p. 187).

The old lawyer's adage of *caveat emptor* (buyer beware) is a useful one for practitioners to adopt, and reflects the healthy scepticism so necessary to critical thinking in adulthood (Brookfield, 1987). If nursing is to truly come of age within this brave new world of twenty-first century health care, then it may have to face some uncomfortable home truths about the cultural values it espouses and then (according to accounts emerging from this study) fails to deliver to a significant number of its practitioners.

Contemplating the rubble: emotions and the research process

Having negotiated the data mountain, the final section of this chapter is intended to highlight the issue of the emotional involvement of coresearchers in the research process. This concerns expectations surrounding the research process, and the estimated effects of the study on its participants and others affected by it.

Qualitative researchers are said to gain control of their projects only by first allowing themselves to lose it (Kleinman *et al.*, 1992, p. 9). In popular research mythology, 'the researcher becomes the hero who went on a dangerous journey and lived to tell us about it' (Kleinman & Copp, 1993, p. 17). Emotions and research from a positivist point of view could be seen as a straightforward contradiction in terms. The emotional involvement of researchers in their fieldwork receives scant and dismissive attention in the research literature, with the notable exceptions generally being found in the feminist canon.

For this particular researcher and the scores of fieldworkers who entered into the study, emotions represented two sides of a rather weathered coin. The first side concerned the emotions generated by the study of a new role learning (an emotional subject, it appears, in its own right), while the second represented the emotions which surfaced as a result of being involved in a collaborative research project where the stakeholders were the researchers themselves. If the project failed, then we could all expect to take a share in the disappointment. If the project succeeded, then we could all anticipate taking some of the credit. Such is the basis on which an action research study of this nature is based.

When considering the rubble left after the substantial period of digging, drilling and sifting through the mass of data acquired, it is important to reflect on the emotional aftermath of the project, as undoubtedly there were both costs and benefits to be had from a lengthy, demanding and searching study. One of the challenges associated with all research concerns *validity*, i.e. whether it did what it really claimed to do, and whether the results are to be believed (McNiff, 1988, p. 131).

Claims to validity

McNiff describes several steps towards establishing the validity of a claim to knowledge, beginning with *self and peer validation*. Certain criteria may be used to judge an individual's claim to knowledge. An educational enquiry in her view begins with a declaration of values, and the desire to turn a negative state into a positive one. Critical reflection, as the way in which naïve understanding is transformed into something more meaningful, is necessary to the project, as is the researchers' ability to 'demonstrate publicly' that systematic, disciplined enquiry has been followed in order to arrive at any hypotheses formed. Peer validation requires a public examination of 'claims to know': the ethic of peer validation is to engage in dialogue, so that dialogue means the sharing of a particular discourse.

The emotional investment required of this study was high. In achieving its stated aims, an in-depth and sometimes emotionally painful investigation of the feelings and values about human nature and human interaction was necessary. In examining critical incidents, for example, the issues discussed ranged from witnessing patients bleeding to death, to allowing someone to die, to caring for the severely disabled and disturbed, to feeling in turn needed and rejected by the system which by all accounts and purposes exists to deliver humane care.

While some co-researchers devised ways of protecting themselves emotionally from the most searching questions, (for example, some participants chose to share a 'stock' or partially invented critical incident, rather than expose themselves to peer scrutiny and discussion over their actions), others were prepared to make much more startling disclosures. The primary researcher's increasing unease at such disclosures was alleviated by the empathy and gentleness of those listening: by the extraordinary experience of having nurses come together to discuss their most heartfelt concerns and memories, and by their colleagues' careful and considered responses to what included information which – outside of the metaphorical four walls of the study – could be considered a legal and ethical minefield. What was clear is that practitioners found talking and sharing and empathising with each other a new and (for some) redefining experience.

The protection of researcher confidentiality is an assumed one in the literature, with few signposts being provided for the unwitting researcher delving into unknown, and largely uncharted, territory. There must have been times when co-researchers were shocked by disclosures, or occasions when revulsion against certain attitudes or stances must have challenged their abilities to be polite, to understand and to overcome personal prejudices.

For some nurses, the study clearly represented the first 'safe' opportunity they had had for sharing their anguish or misery over a certain issue. The possibility of 'emotional contagion' or 'postural echo', where individuals feel compelled to share in others' anger, frustration, pleasure or distress, must therefore have been, on reflection, an ever-present one (see Hatfield *et al.*, 1994). The feelings generated called for a high degree of personal tolerance.

However, given the negativity and derision expressed by participants regarding the support of their colleagues, the reality remained that within the safe space of the study they were still able to maintain a sense of mutual respect and candour about the 'reality shock' of nursing work without placing themselves in a morally difficult position. This came as a genuine and life-affirming surprise to many participants, as is evident in the comments which were received on formal evaluations of the process. Whether this 'safe space' still exists, or whether anyone now regrets their disclosure, remains a matter of open conjecture. The opportunity still exists for researchers to remain collaborative, and to maintain supportive collegiality. Whether they will is ultimately their decision.

Expectations of the research process were also extremely high. For the primary researcher this caused particular difficulties in that the study was interpreted as promising much more than could realistically be attained. Coming as it did in the wake of major organisational reforms, the opportunity to shape and manage transitions through the project was occasionally interpreted as a means for managing structural change more effectively. Thus staff who anticipated a positive career move and who were then offered only redundancy perhaps suffered more emotionally because of the study's involvement than they might have done had it never existed.

Although this remains on the researcher's conscience, in reality there were forces operating outside the study which at the beginning were perhaps too dimly realised by all concerned. At the very least the study can be said to have acquired culturally valid answers to the research questions posed.

Kleinman and Copp are critical of the belief that talking to others about problems or uncertainties in research makes us vulnerable to charges of incompetence or weakness. They urge researchers to acknowledge instead their '*inter*dependence' with the outside world. By claiming the strengths (and presumably) weaknesses of our methods and the uniqueness of our identity, we will in the end make better fieldworkers. It is, they say, possible to recognise the constructed nature of our work without 'having it muddy our critical eye':

> 'We can give up the individualist model and instead create inter-disciplinary networks and informal groups that encourage us to give and receive intellectual and emotional support. In our experience, having co-operative contexts in which to think, talk and write makes us work better and feel better.'

> (Kleinman & Copp, 1993, pp. 56–7)

The clarification of values inherent in an occupational culture may well help individuals to increase their motivation and sense of belonging at work, or in the mutual sharing of different world views within a social situation. Hence, while it is not suggested that the findings of this study can be generalised to any particular population, generalisation to the theory itself may indeed be possible across a broad spectrum of occupations and life experiences.

We perhaps do a disservice to learners when we allow them to imagine that there is such a thing as order in the world, and that someone, somewhere will take responsibility for making it happen. The provisional nature of human experience, and the emotional crisis inflicted by this dishonesty, are perhaps things which require emotional courage to accept. Whatever our personal feelings about our stake in the future, learners have a right to relate and deal with the insecurities and uncertainties of their past. This need does not go away when they join the professional register.

The criteria for providing effective preceptorship formulated by co-researchers in this study can be adopted by practitioners of any specialism (see Fig. 3.1). Our experience of using and developing our own practice-based model of preceptorship would suggest that it is indeed flexible, and that the opportunities for making this happen may be greater than we have previously realised.

In striving towards a practice based theory of preceptorship, four criteria appear to be cardinal in managing effective and personally sustaining learning transitions:

(1) Formal support mechanisms require the strategic and committed support of those managing organisations, whether in the workplace or in the delivery of educational opportunity.

(2) Values clarification between the experienced and the inexperienced is a necessary and valuable prerequisite to acquiring the skills and emotional literacy required to negotiate the transition from novice to confident practitioner.

(3) Expectations of the beginning practitioner must be made explicit, or the will to succeed may be compromised by confusion and 'interpersonal moral distress'. Realistic but positively constructed appraisal of what is expected of the newcomer is preferable to a rosy interpretation which then leaves the individual feeling inadequate and 'out of step' with their new colleagues.

(4) Attempts to create a culturally permissible 'safe space' which allows for the testing and formulation of self-concept in relation to new work has potentially significant advantages for the employer as well as the employee. This enables expectations of the new employee to be properly and meaningfully articulated, resulting in fewer misapprehensions and errors in decision-making, both personally and in relation to the achievement of organisational goals. The greater the level of clarification, the less dissatisfaction and dissonance is expressed.

Fig. 3.1 Criteria for providing effective preceptorship.

The future of preceptorship policy: could it become a statutory requirement?

Opportunities to extend preceptorship to other areas of practice and occupational territories remain a vital consideration for policymakers. Within nursing itself the case for making preceptor support a statutory requirement has already been highlighted (Maben & Macleod-Clark, 1997a). Our study would certainly confirm that a formal period of preceptor support based on principles similar to our own is an extremely valuable means of improving awareness of professional accountability, while at the same time recognising its limitations. The power of preceptorship to bring about collegiality and a sense of mutuality and trust in the workplace and to transform it into a 'high trust' environment is profound, and would greatly enhance any attempts to bolster recruitment and retention practice and entice returners back into the professions.

An important caveat to this, however, is that preceptorship (and thus professional learning support) only works when support for its aims exists at all levels of the hierarchy and in all reaches of the organisation. Take away support at any level and the resource and its positive impact will simply fade away.

Career transitions are commonplace, as the literature amply testifies (e.g. Zapf, 1991; Kachoyeanos-Selder, 1993; Knox, 1995). The potential to identify the transitional learning needs of other staff in both public and private sector occupations is virtually unlimited. Police, ambulance, paramedic and fire service personnel, social workers, doctors, academics, student counsellors, teachers, probation officers and professional therapists of all hues, all stand to benefit from the sense of personal control brought about by improved emotional literacy. Emotion is in the end integral to all human experience.

Education and learning have both the potential to change the world and to alter perspectives on the right way to live. If, as educators, we are to encourage 'teaching as care' so that as Plato advised, 'those having torches will pass them on to others' (Daloz, 1986, p. 236), we will have to remain sensitive and proactive in seeing that in future what we espouse as professionals is also what we *do*. Only then will we be able to say with confidence that we 'care' professionally.

Appendix: The Socratic method

Born the son of an Athenian stonemason in 469 BC, the philosopher Socrates became disillusioned with the ignorance and apparent complacency of the politicians and sages of his time, believing (unlike his predecessors) that virtue could not be taught, but rather could only come from a systematic examination of our human values.

He developed a form of dialogue known as 'the elenchus', a systematic 'examination of life' through dialogue. Socrates did not profess to be a teacher or a leader, but saw himself and others as 'fellow seekers after truth'. Essentially, he questioned people about what they thought they knew. He invented a method of questioning which sought to analyse and clarify the meaning of fundamental value terms. By patient questioning and examination of opinion for its logical consequences, Socrates sought consistency in fundamental definitions of meaning.

Even when opinions are thought to be correct, he asserted, they need to be further supported by a principled account of why it is believed and must be so. Successful 'elenchus' or dialogue then is thought to increase our collective stock of true beliefs by finding answers to those important questions which have practical implications for the everyday conduct of our lives. In examining practitioners' views of transitional learning support in the preceptorship study discussed in Chapter 3, co-researchers were asked to examine their values and beliefs about what it means to be a beginner in nursing, and about the nature of support that 'ought' or 'should' be provided to preceptees in the early stages of their careers.

Once agreement had been reached about the situation which already existed, i.e. the current support offered (or not, as the case may be!) the questions raised were, 'is this enough?' and 'could it be done better, differently, more sensitively and if so, how and why?'. Socrates' most important principle was, 'Is this the right way to live?', and through the use of focus group methodology and skilful facilitation, groups can begin to ask these vital questions. As one person makes a statement of their opinion, another person may refute it or argue against it, while at the same time being asked to justify their position. The group concludes a discussion on a particular theme when they are satisfied that the position they have adopted is consistent, meaningful, justifiable and fair, given their situation and other demands made on them.

Further reading on Socratic dialogue

Carlton, E. (1995) *Values and the Social Sciences – an Introduction*. Duckworth, London.
This is a good introduction to ideas about values education and values clarification generally.

Ferre, F. (1996) *Being and Value: a Constructive Postmodern Metaphysics.* SUNY Press, New York.
This rather weighty book is very rewarding in that it takes quite difficult philosophical concepts and makes them seem straightforward. The author is an enthusiast and it shows!

Jordan, W. (1990) *Ancient Concepts of Philosophy.* Routledge, London.
Another helpful introductory text which places Socratic thought into historical context.

Livingstone, R.W. (1935) *Greek Ideals and Modern Life.* Oxford University Press, Oxford.
Worth taking the time to find through inter-library loan, this book helps to relate philosophy to the basic questions of human existence, showing that little has actually changed in society, millennium or no!

Perkinson, H.J. (1989) *Since Socrates – Studies in the History of Western Educational Thought.* Longman, New York.
This is an excellent and enlightening read for educationalists in that the reader is able to see where modern politicians get their (sometimes!) antiquated ideas about learning from. It is truly humbling to see that ideas discussed three millennia ago are still cherished today.

Saunders, T.J., translation of Plato (1987) *Early Socratic Dialogues.* Penguin, London.
All we know of Socrates we obtain from the writings of Plato. Socrates was so reviled in his time he was sentenced to be executed, although he drank the famous draught of hemlock and died before he could be made the public spectacle his enemies dreamed about. These dialogues are the purest form of Socratic dialogue we have, and the translator provides very helpful commentary to help us place the method into historical and contemporary contexts.

Seeskin, K. (1987) *Dialogue and Discovery – a Study in Socratic Method.* SUNY Press, New York.
This was the serendipitous find which inspired the present author to undertake Socratic method in the first place. It is a truly clever and incisive guide to understanding the meaning and aims of Socrates' dialogue. If you only have time to read one book on Socrates then this is the one which will help you most, particularly if you are keen to try out the method in your own workplace.

References

Allanach, B. (1988) Interviewing to evaluate preceptorship relationships. *Journal of Nursing Staff Development*, Fall issue, 152–7.
Bain, L. (1996) Preceptorship: a review of the literature. *Journal of Advanced Nursing*, **24**, 104–7.
Benner, P. & Benner, R.V. (1979) *The New Nurses' Work Entry – a Troubled Sponsorship.* Tiresias Press, New York.

Bowles, N. (1995) A critical appraisal of preceptorship. *Nursing Standard*, **9** (35), 25–8.

Brookfield, S.D. (1987) *Developing Critical Thinkers: Challenging Adults to Explore New Ways of Thinking and Acting.* Open University Press, Milton Keynes.

Brykczynska, G. (1993) Nursing values: nightmares and nonsense. In: *Nursing: Its Hidden Agendas,* (eds M. Jolley & G. Brykczynska), pp. 131–158. Chapman & Hall, London.

Boyle, D.K., Popkess-Vawter, S. & Taunton, R.L. (1996) Socialization of new graduate nurses in critical care. *Heart-Lung,* **25** (2), 141–54.

Burman, E. (1994) *Deconstructing Developmental Psychology.* Routledge, London.

Casey, C. (1995) *Work, Self and Society.* Routledge, London.

Chalmers, H. (1995) Accountability in nursing models and the nursing process. pp. 33–48. In: *Accountability in Nursing Practice,* (ed. R. Watson). Chapman & Hall, London.

Coates, V.E. & Gormley, E. (1997) Learning the practice of nursing: views about preceptorship. *Nurse Education Today,* 17, 91–8.

Daloz, L.A. (1986) *Effective Teaching and Mentoring: Realizing the Transformational Power of Adult Learning Experiences.* Jossey-Bass, San Francisco.

Davies, C. (1995) *Gender and the Professional Predicament in Nursing.* Open University Press, Buckingham.

Dimond, B. (1994) Legal aspects of role expansion. In: *Expanding the Role of the Nurse: the Scope of Professional Practice,* (eds G. Hunt & P. Wainwright). Blackwell Science, Oxford.

DoH (1991) *The Patients' Charter,* HMSO, London.

DoH (1995) *The Patients' Charter and You.* HMSO, London.

Dwivedi, K.N. (ed.) (1997). *The Therapeutic Use of Stories,* Routledge, London.

Dwivedi, K.N. & Gardner, D. (1997) Theoretical perspectives and clinical approaches. In: *The Therapeutic Use of Stories,* (ed. K.N. Dwivedi) pp. 19–41. Routledge, London.

Ellis, H. (1992) Conceptions of care. In: *Themes and Perspectives in Nursing,* (eds K. Soothill, C. Henry & K. Kendrick), pp. 196–213. Chapman & Hall, London.

Farmer, B. (1993) The Use and Abuse of Power in Nursing. *Nursing Standard,* **7** (23), 33–5.

Fineman, S. & Gabriel, Y. (1996) *Experiencing Organisations.* Sage, London.

Flanagan, H. & Spurgeon, P. (1996) *Public Sector Managerial Effectiveness: Theory and Practice in the National Health Service.* Open University Press, Buckingham.

Fleck, E. & Fyffe, T. (1997) Changing nursing practice through continuing education: a tool for evaluation. *Journal of Nursing Management,* **5**, 37–41.

Goldenberg, D., Iwasiw, C. & McMaster, E. (1997) Self-efficacy of senior baccalaureate nursing students and preceptors. *Nurse Education Today,* 17, 303–10.

Hardey, M. (1994) The dissemination and utilization of nursing research. In: *Nursing Research – Theory and Practice*, (eds M. Hardey & A. Mulhall), pp. 163–85. Chapman & Hall, London.

Hatfield, E. Cacioppo, J.T. Rapson, R.L. (1994) *Emotional Contagion*. Editions de la Maison des Sciences de l'Homme/Cambridge University Press, Paris.

Hewitt, J.P. (1994) *Self and Society – a Symbolic Interactionist Social Psychology*, Allyn & Bacon, Boston.

Hochschild, A.R. (1979) Emotion work, feeling rules and social structure. *American Journal of Sociology*, **85**, 551–75.

Hochschild, A.R. (1983) *The Managed Heart*. University of California Press, Berkeley.

Kachoyeanos-Selder, M. (1993) Death and Dying – Life Transitions of Parents at the Unexpected Death of a School-age and Older Child. *Journal of Paediatric Nursing*, **8** (1), 41–9.

Kapborg, I.D. & Fischbein, S. (1998) Nurse Education and Professional Work: Transition Problems? *Nurse Education Today*, **18**, 165–71.

Kleinman, S. & Copp, M.A. (1993) *Emotions and fieldwork*. A Sage University Paper, Qualitative Research Methods Series 28. Sage, Newbury Park.

Kleinman, S., Copp, M.A. & Henderson, K. (1992) *Qualitatively Different: Teaching Field Work to Graduate Students*, manuscript submitted for publication, mentioned in Kleinman & Copp (1993), p. 65.

Knox, S.N. (1995) Career transitions of the nurse executive in the United States. *Nursing Administration Quarterly*, **19** (4), 62–70.

Kramer, M. (1974) *Reality Shock: Why Nurses Leave Nursing*. Mosby, St Louis.

Maben, J. & Macleod-Clark, J. (1997a) The impact of project 2000. NT Occasional Paper. *Nursing Times*, **93** (35), 55–8.

Maben, J. & Macleod-Clark, J. (1997b) *Project 2000: Perceptions of the Philosophy and Practice of Nursing*. ENB Study. English National Board, London.

MacIntyre, A. (1985) *After Virtue*, (2nd edn.) University of Notre Dame Press, Paris.

McNiff, J. (1988) *Action Research: Principles & Practice*. Routledge, London.

Morton-Cooper, A. (1992) *An evaluation of preceptorship as an appropriate conceptual model for British continuing nurse education*. MEd dissertation, University of Warwick.

Morton-Cooper, A. (1993) *Working definitions for preceptorship*. Confidential regional health authority discussion paper.

Morton-Cooper, A. (1998) *Preceptorship via action research: a reflective account*. Doctoral thesis, University of Warwick.

Morton-Cooper, A. (2000 in press) *Action Research in Health Care*. Blackwell Science, Oxford.

Mullin, J. (1996) Down, on the Farm. *The Guardian*, 10 January, Suppl. p. 3.

Norr, K. F. (1994) Using quantitative and qualitative methods to assess impact on practice. In: *Disseminating Research/Changing Practice*, Research Methods for Primary Care, (eds E.V. Dunn, P.G. Norton, M. Stewart, F. Tudiver & M.J. Bass), vol.6. Sage, Thousand Oaks, California.

Sarbin, R.R. & Kitsuse, J.I. (eds) (1994) *Constructing the Social.* Sage, London.

Savage, J. (1995) *Nursing Intimacy – an Ethnographic Approach to Nurse-Patient Interaction.* Scutari Press, London.

Scott, P.A. (1995) Role, Role Enactment and the Health Care Practitioner. *Journal of Advanced Nursing,* **2** (2), 323–8.

Sloan, T. (1996) *Damaged Life: the Crisis of the Modern Psyche.* Routledge, London.

Smith, P. (1992) *The Emotional Labour of Nursing.* Macmillan, Basingstoke.

UKCC (1993) *Registrar's Letter: the Council's Position Concerning a Period of Support and Preceptorship: Implementation of the Post-Registration Education and Practice Project Proposals.* UKCC, London.

UKCC (1996) *Guidelines for Professional Practice.* UKCC, London.

UKCC (1999) *Fitness for Practice,* the report of the UKCC Commission for Nursing and Midwifery Education. UKCC, London.

Zapf, M.K. (1991) Cross-cultural transitions and wellness: dealing with culture shock. *International Journal for the advancement of Counselling,* **14** (2), 105–19.

Further reading

Work design and job strain

Brykczynska, G. (1995) Reflective practice: an analysis of nursing wisdom. In *Nursing: Beyond Tradition and Conflict,* (eds M. Jolley & G. Brykczynska) pp. 9–28. Mosby, London.

Collinson, D. (1994) Strategies of resistance: power, knowledge and subjectivity in the workplace. In: *Resistance and Power in Organisations,* (eds J.M. Jernier, D. Knights & W.R. Nord), pp. 25–68. Routledge, London.

Corwin, R.G. (1961) Role conception and career aspiration: a study of identity in nursing. *Social Quarterly,* **2,** 69–86.

Greenwood, J. (1993) The apparent desensitization of student nurses during their professional socialization: a cognitive perspective. *Journal of Advanced Nursing,* **18,** 1471–9.

Karasek, R.A. Jr. (1979) Job demands, job decision latitude and mental strain, implications for job redesign. *Administrative Science Quarterly,* **24,** 285–308.

Koslowsky, M. (1998) *Modelling the Stress–Strain Relationship in Work Settings.* Routledge, London/New York.

Krausz, M., Koslowsky, M., Shalom, N. & Elkayim, N. (1995) prediction of intention to leave the ward, the hospital, and the nursing profession: a longitudinal study. *Journal of Organizational Behaviour,* **16,** 277–88.

Newell, S. (1995) *The Healthy Organization: Fairness, Ethics and Effective Management.* Routledge, London.

Newton, T., Handy, J. & Fineman, S. (1995) 'Managing' Stress: Emotion and Power at Work. Sage, London.

Sennett, R. (1998) *The Corrosion of Character: the Personal Consequences of Work in the New Capitalism*. W.W. Norton & Co, New York.

Social support

Cobb, S. (1976) Social support as a mediator of life stress. *Psychosomatic Medicine*, **38** (5), 300–14.
Dean, A. (1977) The stress buffering role of social support – problems and prospects for systematic investigation. *The Journal of Nervous and Mental Disease*, **165** (6), 403–17.
Dewe, P.J. & Guest, D.E. (1990) Methods of coping with stress at work: a conceptual analysis and empirical study of measurement issues. *Journal of Organizational Behavior*, **11**, 135–150.
Jackson, I. (1997) Coping with stress. *Nursing Times*, **93** (29), 31–2.
Stoter, D. (1997) *Staff Support in Health Care*. Blackwell Science, Oxford.

Emotional literacy

Lazarus, R.S. (1991) *Emotions and Adaptation*. Oxford University Press, Oxford/New York.
Orbach, S. (1994) *What's Really Going on Here? Making Sense of Our Emotional Lives*. Virago Press, London.

Researching your own practice

Rolfe, G. (1998) *Expanding Nursing Knowledge: Understanding and Researching Your Own Practice*. Butterworth-Heinemann, Oxford.

Improving your personal influencing skills

Gillen, T. (1995) *Positive Influencing Skills*. Institute of Personnel & Development, London.
Hale, R. & Whitlam, P. (1995) *The Power of Personal Influence*. McGraw Hill Book Company, Maidenhead.

Chapter 4
Clinical Supervision: Making the Connections

'Clinical supervision is still a delicate seedling. If we don't protect it, it may shrivel and die, or flourish in a few special environments only – like so many other nursing innovations of the last decade.'

Jane Salvage

Introduction

It is interesting to note that when we reflected on the contents for the first edition, we focused our attention primarily on mentoring and preceptorship because at that time these support relationships were actively being explored in nursing and the wider health care arena. Mentoring had been suggested as a suitable support relationship for student nurses, and preceptorship was emerging in a modified form from its original North American interpretations, as appropriate for newly qualified nurses, midwives and health visitors. We readily acknowledge that, when writing the first edition, our personal and academic interests concerned developing our ideas around these two emerging relationships and that our more pragmatic selves were interested in discovering how they could be applied appropriately to clinical practice.

Having drawn Philip Burnard's attention to mentoring in 1987 and having assisted the English National Board (ENB) in its considerations, the scene was set for further deliberations on professional support roles and relationships that still excite some six years on (Palmer, 1987; Burnard, 1988; ENB, 1988; Morton-Cooper, 1998). However, the clinical support scene has continued to change, particularly in nursing, and clinical supervision has become a significant factor in the continuing professional support debate. The time has therefore come to reflect on clinical supervision and to begin to make the relevant connections with the other main professional support roles of mentoring and preceptor-ship, as well as to explore the relevant education strategies and approaches that affect the provision of meaningful, support relation-ships in practice.

Perhaps if we had focused less on our 'respectable passions', we would have entered the debate concerning clinical supervision at an earlier stage. However, with the calls for collaborative practice and new quality initiatives, the time is right to join the critical discourse con-cerning this significant professional support relationship – a relationship that enables support, professional development and a critical space where practitioners can examine their practice and the quality of care that they provide.

The deliberations for this last part of the book are built on the authors' experiences of working with groups of staff throughout the health service and in higher education, and of implementing and evaluating support frameworks. Our work with doctors and GPs has mostly involved preparation for mentoring, while nurses, midwives and health visitors have been concerned with the introduction of clinical super-vision and preceptorship in primary and secondary care.

The intention of this chapter is to explore clinical supervision as it is currently developing in nursing practice, and within the literature, allowing us to make connections between the other significant support relationships in practice. The resulting discussions will include attempts at identifying the origins of clinical supervision and will centre around the sharing of good practice to encourage others to engage in supportive relationships of this type. What is required is not a continual reframing of the debate but a critical dialogue concerning the needs and requirements of those nurses and health care practitioners who will be expected to engage in some form of clinical supervision in the future (DoH, 1993; UKCC, 1996; J.M. Consulting Ltd, 1998).

This dialogue is particularly necessary and relevant now that initiatives are underway for the arrival of new quality strategies and procedures (DoH, 1999). Our discussions will be mindful that the rationale for providing appropriate support and development is an important aspect of service delivery. Modern organisations are complex and demanding and the NHS is no exception, but it is essential to remember that the patient, client or user is the central focus for this service.

In this chapter we will also identify the other support relationships, such as peer learning, coaching and personal tutoring, and will explore the nature of supervision and learning support for those new to a pro-fession or occupation – the student. This is undertaken to assist prac-titioners, managers and educators to make informed decisions in selecting and implementing appropriate support frameworks, as there remains some confusion in roles and how these are interpreted in practice (Wilson-Barnett *et al.*, 1995; Cahill, 1996; White, 1996).

Reflections of the past

A variety of key roles have previously been identified in providing professional learning support for students in clinical placements, for the newly qualified, and for the experienced practitioner wanting to make sense of his/her world of practice. These roles have been instrumental in developing practitioners for the professional working world, and particularly in social work and occupational therapy, supervisors have responsibilities for assisting learning and clinical socialisation.

In nursing, midwifery and health visiting the roles of clinical supervisors, field work practice teachers, clinical teachers, assessors and latterly mentors have been established to enhance learning and provide learning support as previously discussed. The prevailing emphasis was placed on the application of supervision and clinical teaching to prepare students, and provide role models for practice (Orton, 1981; Ogier, 1989).

In the past, supervision in areas of general nursing had become too specifically focused on mainly punitive, monitoring elements (Tichen & Binnie, 1995). Nursing researchers report the dissatisfaction with supervision but were positive in suggesting that:

> 'supportive, competent supervision is essential if nurses are to give their best to the care of the ill, frail and vulnerable.'

> (Ogier & Cameron-Buccheri, 1990, p. 24)

As a result of the past difficulties and negative connotations associated with supervision, new roles were formulated, particularly for student groups, as curriculum planning was under way during the early stages of Project 2000 implementation (UKCC, 1986). In social work, mental health and the other therapies it is traditionally the supervisor who provides a supportive and critical space for another professional practitioner who commonly is referred to as the supervisee. However, in nursing a variety of terms have developed for such a relationship as attempts were made to adapt traditional approaches of supervision from the other professional groups and health care occupations. Such terms as coach or facilitator, and given the sensitivity of the culture in some clinical areas and the scepticism concerning the relationship, labels such as clinical supporter and coach have been variously used to denote a clinical supervisory relationship. Nurses involved in a pilot study to implement clinical supervision selected clinical supporter as a suitable term for the role of supervisor to differentiate this role from the preponderance of other roles that had blossomed in their particular clinical arena. It was also found that clinical supervision had a negative meaning for them at this time, (Palmer & Wilson, 1997).

There is continued evidence that despite the plethora of information nurses remain reluctant and sceptical about engaging in clinical supervision for a variety of organisational, educational and personal reasons (McEvoy, 1993; McCallion & Baxter, 1995; Wright *et al.*, 1997; Wilson & Palmer, 1998). This is supported in a report which identified that fewer than 50% of district nurses in one particular study had any clinical supervision within the last year (Audit Commission, 1999).

A common question asked in our workshops on clinical supervision and when establishing clinical support frameworks in practice is, 'What is clinical supervision'? Despite the many accessible articles, worthwhile texts and policy statements there remains a conviction that practitioners still have limited understanding, and that for them to fully comprehend and appreciate the virtues of clinical supervision, they need to experience it for themselves (Bond & Holland, 1998). However, if they retain negative views of supervision/clinical supervision it becomes probable that they will not make strenuous attempts to undertake such experience.

It is our view in working with practitioners from a variety of healthcare settings that practitioners are still not readily embracing or experiencing clinical supervision. We believe that it is still viewed, in some areas, with suspicion because:

- There remains a prevailing sense that it is being imposed 'top–down' and is not supported by managerial commitment
- Nurses in primary and secondary care settings (less so in mental health) remain sceptical about management's involvement in the relationship and process
- The terminology in some of the models and frameworks has not been interpreted or has not 'travelled' well from the original authors' deliberations, resulting in lack of understanding and appreciation of the original ideas
- There is a misguided perception, but a frequently rehearsed one, that practitioners are already carrying out clinical supervision: 'We are already doing it and have been for years' (Wilson & Palmer, 1999)
- The links between the need for professional support and in particular clinical supervision, with other recently introduced activities of the 'reflective practitioner', portfolio building and continual learning in practice have not been readily translated into practice.

Addressing such perceptions, misinterpretations, fears and lack of understanding forms a vital part of the process of assisting practitioners to come to terms with clinical supervision in practice. By confronting anxieties and correcting misunderstandings, practitioners can help themselves deal with the relevant issues surrounding this important professional support role. If practitioners can begin to make sense of the rich pattern of their experiences and start to make the necessary connections with the requirements for continual learning and updating in practice, then the need for appropriate supervision activities will become apparent.

Such issues will be discussed within the following headings: decoding clinical supervision; the current context of clinical supervision; and making clinical supervision work. At the end of the chapter a section of common questions asked by participants in workshops and seminars and when we are out and about in practice, will draw in relevant practical issues concerning clinical supervision and its implementation.

To make sense of clinical supervision and the relevant connections with practice it is important to appreciate the history, language, tensions and challenges, as clinical supervision has developed from its origins within other professions or occupational groups and is currently being translated in nursing.

Decoding supervision and clinical supervision

There are a wide range of worthwhile texts and articles that explore supervision in depth from differing occupational perspectives, (Hawkins & Shohet, 1989; Pritchard, 1995). Others thoughtfully introduce its nursing counterpart, 'clinical' supervision', and make useful connections with supervision in health and social care, as well as offering practical solutions and effective preparation for making clinical supervision a viable proposition in nursing (Butterworth & Faugier, 1992; Bishop, 1998; Bond & Holland, 1998; Butterworth *et al.*, 1998; Open University, 1998). However there is not universal approval and Wolsey and Leach (1997) raise interesting questions about conceptual flaws and the financial burden of implementing clinical supervision. Financial reasons are also cited for not making clinical supervision a statutory requirement throughout the NHS in the 1998 statutory body review (J.M. Consulting Ltd, 1998).

To fully appreciate clinical supervision in its richness and diversity, it is perhaps sensible to tease out the meaning and interpretations of supervision from its traditional roots, before adaptations are made for its transfer to the nursing, midwifery and health visiting setting. This is important if those practitioners who may ultimately benefit from such relationships are to accept and own the supervisory process, and make useful comparisons with the other professional support roles that currently exist.

Supervision, or 'traditional supervision' as we have identified the original concept in order to separate it clearly from its nursing counterpart of clinical supervision, is taken here to mean supervisory relationships as practised and developed by a range of professional and occupational groups other than general nursing. Supervisory relationships concern what others have identified as the enabling and ensuring aspects of effecting a positive developmental relationship that ensures accountability, as well as enabling support and individual development (Kadushin, 1976; Proctor, 1986).

Such relationships are now seen as positive and enabling and do not appear to bear the negative connotations that affect this intriguing concept when it is transferred to general nursing practice. Although initially there were tensions evident in seeking an appropriate equilibrium of the enabling and ensuring aspects, as will be discussed later, these appear to have mostly been resolved by social work, counselling and the therapy disciplines.

For several decades trainers in the field of youth and community work have traditionally developed supervisory relationships working with students and practitioners to help them 'enrich understanding and gain the skills needed to bring theory and practice within a coherent and workable whole' (Marchant, 1986, p. 37). Significant relationships were formed between a supervisor and supervisee (or in our case the preferred term is that of practitioner), working in partnership to facilitate learning from experience and the gaining of new skills, as well as the ownership of new knowledge through making the connections with existing concepts and constructs. Such relationships were provided for workers at all levels of development, from those experienced in practice to those being introduced to the field of practice.

Prins (cited Marchant, 1986)), in classifying the 'ensuring and enabling aspects' of supervision, had laid the foundation for many of the deliberations and models that seek to strike a coherent balance between the management and developmental functions of supervision for social workers, trainers and therapists. This set the scene for the tensions and challenges that can arise in seeking an appropriate balance between the ensuring and enabling functions. Westheimer (1977) and Marchant (1986) make helpful contributions in continuing the discourse concerning the nature of supervision and by exploring how the various health and therapy disciplines have traditionally struggled to come to terms with the inherent tensions of such relationships.

Marchant (1986) interprets the ensuring function of supervision as that of 'getting the job done', and links this to the term 'management supervision'. This may mean that there is a clear management component identified within the supervisory processes or that the relationship is one which fits with the organisational structures. Other authors identify differing struggles and write of the uncomfortable 'piggy in the middle' position within traditional supervisory approaches, with resulting tensions between management accountability and professional responsibility (Hughes & Pengelly, 1997).

Supervisors who are also line managers is the situation more readily found in mental health and learning disabilities arenas where the tendency is for all staff to engage in supervision and managers have a clear role in the process. Well defined boundaries are imperative for this type of supervision relationship, but it may not be so easily acceptable to general nursing, still addressing a history of occupational strategies and professional predicaments (Davies, 1976; Davies, 1995).

Marchant (1986) also identifies another type of supervision he categorises as 'independent supervision', which is a type of supervision that is freer of organisational influences but one that may still be affected by organisational pressures and constraints. Independent supervision provides the enabling function of assisting practitioners to learn from their experiences and develop practice expertise, independent from managerial intervention. However, as he readily admits, it is not quite as straightforward as this categorisation into the two types of supervision would reflect.

He acknowledges that in the literature and in practice, independent supervision can also be referred to as consultancy, professional supervision or non-managerial supervision. Marchant is a helpful source in interpreting supervision categories, (what form it takes) and style (how it is carried out). Styles of supervision, and these are recognisable within the clinical supervision context, are individual, group, peer or interpersonal, commonly referred to in nursing as types of supervision. These will be explored later in this chapter in the section relating to practitioners' common concerns.

The categories of supervision interpreted from Marchant's and others' deliberations offer an insight into the complexities of supervision and add weight to Brigid Proctor's comment that, 'supervision is one of those irritating words that hold a particular meaning for certain people and quite different associations for others' (Proctor, 1986, p. 23). The other significant categories of supervision that exist are the following:

Tutorial supervision – This essentially provides a tutorial role where the supervisor explores the practitioner's work and care of patients/clients but has no responsibilities for the work being carried out in practice. There is a tutor and student focus with identified supervisor functions of facilitating learning and educating. The linking role with nursing is that of the personal tutor with a balance of enabling elements.

Training supervision – This relates to students in practice or on placements, where the supervisor is expected to have some responsibility for the students' work with patients/clients. There is a trainer and trainee focus, with identified supervisor functions of management and monitoring. The linking roles are those of clinical teacher or lecturer–practitioner, within a balance of ensuring and enabling elements.

Consultancy or professional supervision – This is identified for qualified practitioners responsible for their own case load or practice. There is a consultant and professional practitioner focus with identified supervision functions relating to the offering of support, guidance and advice. The linking role is that of mentoring with a primary focus of enabling rather than ensuring elements.

Peer supervision – This is a relationship of peers resulting in a mutually beneficial relationship where practice issues can be shared and explored. The participants have no direct responsibility for each other's practice and the focus is that of colleague and colleague within a partnership that is supportive, provides feedback and encourages learning. The linking role is that of preceptorship or co-tutoring. (The former has been extensively explored in Chapter 3 while the latter is defined in the glossary of professional support roles in Chapter 5.)

Figure 4.1 shows a family tree of supervisory approaches and illustrates where clinical supervision fits as the current debate unfolds. Here the categories of supervision are laid out to demonstrate their relative connections and enabling and ensuring emphasis, or balance of tasks, demonstrating the primary focus for each particular category. Clinical supervision appears to fall within the enabling aspect but may well have some ensuring or monitoring function when linked specifically to quality assurance. This will be discussed in more detail later in the chapter.

The essential point is that the main categories of supervision (independent and management) are not synonymous but complementary, and they may overlap in the duties, tasks and responsibilities that are inherent with such relationships. Both categories however have relevance in enabling the individual practitioner to reflect, learn and be supported in practice with confidence, within his/her organisational environment. Providing an appropriate balance of ensuring and enabling

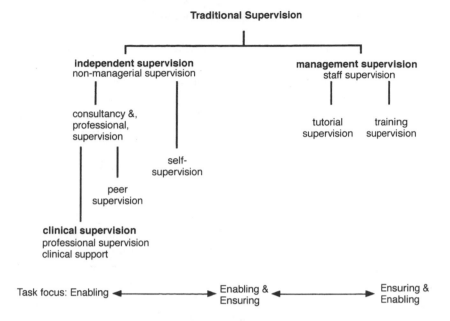

Fig. 4.1 Categories of supervision: a family tree.

duties for effective supervision within such categories requires a degree of skill, empathy and contextual awareness.

It is understandable that social workers were initially suspicious about this type of support relationship, linking it with 'administrative over-seeing' rather then offering management, teaching and enabling components (Westheimer, 1977). Nursing appears to have found itself in a similar situation in seemingly coming to terms with the introduction of clinical supervision, but remaining slightly suspicious and sceptical of its integrity and intent. Perhaps this is a fitting juncture in the discussions to consider the development of clinical supervision as it emerges from its traditional supervision roots and begins to play a significant part in nursing practice.

The current context of clinical supervision

There are those who trace the introduction of clinical supervision in nursing to the findings of the report of the Allitt affair concerning the professional, managerial and organisational incompetence that resulted in the death of several children in a UK hospital (N. Davies, 1993; Bishop, 1994; Clothier *et al.*, 1994). However it is important to note that clinical supervision had been previously identified as playing a significant part in supporting safe practice for community practitioners at a much earlier stage (Butterworth, 1998).

Clinical supervision was highlighted in a strategy for nursing document at about the time of the Clothier Inquiry, in which clinical supervision was considered as a formal professional support and learning process, enabling practitioners to assume responsibility for their own practice as well as enhancing consumer protection and safety of care (DoH, 1993). This offered a clear remit for clinical supervision, and particularly significant in this policy document was the recognition that an essential aspect of such relationships was the encouragement of self-assessment, analytical and reflective skills.

The scene was set with these policy deliberations, the publication of a highly relevant nursing text, statutory body interest and the production of an influential report, for the introduction of clinical supervision to the practice domain (Butterworth & Faugier, 1992; Kohner, 1994; UKCC, 1995; UKCC, 1996). The development of clinical supervision in nursing was clearly focused on a clinical relationship that involves an exchange between professionals, enabling the development of professional skills (Butterworth, 1992). Such relationships enable practitioners and their supervisors to work together to improve practice and increase understanding of professional practice (UKCC, 1996).

As a result of such deliberations an assortment of frameworks and models have been produced and worked on as the discussion about this increasingly important professional support role has continued (Johns, 1993; Farrington, 1995; Nicklin, 1997; Bond & Holland, 1998). The underlying features of most of the conceptual approaches appear to concern maintaining the equilibrium of educative, supportive and clinical elements of such relationships. This is identified in the often quoted aims for the supervision relationship identified by Platt-Koch (1986) which concern:

- Expanding the knowledge base
- Assisting in the development of clinical expertise
- Developing self-esteem and professional autonomy.

A central lynchpin of the emerging conceptual approaches has been the work of Brigid Proctor (1986), and nurse authors in particular have been drawn to her framework of formative, normative and restorative tasks of supervision in devising their own interpretations of clinical supervision. Proctor's seminal work has been interpreted in a variety of ways to advance an understanding of clinical supervision, and to help make sense of this intriguing professional support role. A framework of cooperative accountability is suggested, with supervision as an enabling process that facilitates practitioners to 'develop as an effective working person' within a partnership that focuses on client care. The practitioner works with a supervisor to 'render an account of herself in order to assure herself, and anyone who may be requiring her to be accountable, that she is practising responsibly' (Proctor, 1986, p. 23).

Within such a cooperative relationship there are certain predisposing conditions and values that have to be discussed, shared and implicitly understood. These involve appreciating (Proctor, 1986):

- The nature of competence and effective practice
- That individuals may bring material to the partnership that is 'selectively presented'
- That self-assessment is essential.

This last condition is vital as Inskipp and Proctor (1993) begin to separate the meanings of the enabling and ensuring duties of supervision within the formative, normative and restorative tasks previously explored by Proctor. There is recognition that the enabling, independent supervision relationship has no formal assessment or managerial task.

It is useful to refer back to the original work to fully appreciate Proctor's perspective on taking the clinical supervision debate forward. It would appear that there is a tendency in the nursing literature to relate the differing concepts, tasks and roles underpinning Proctor's original ideas with the earlier deliberations of both Kadushin (1976) and Westheimer (1977). Kadushin prepared the way by identifying the main functions of supervision as being those of an educative, supportive and managerial nature. Westheimer identified within social work supervision the importance of the management, teaching and enabling components of supervisory relationships.

Although such connections and merging of ideas may be helpful initially in gaining an understanding of the intricacies of clinical supervision, there is a concern that the essence of a shared, cooperative relationship, and particularly the restorative tasks, may be gradually diminished and eventually lost. In Proctor's framework this task concerns more than providing basic support as it offers a creative dimension for refreshment and recharging of energies. This provides a vital space for re-examining current situations, producing new ideas and exploring new ways of working – achieved if independent supervision is considered as a cooperative experience, enabling personal and professional accountability.

Nicklin (1995) and Northcott (1998a) offer sound adaptations by making links between Proctor's deliberations and the managerial, educative and supportive modes that could be seen to be readily applicable to nursing and health care. Others such as the Chief Nursing Officer (1994) and Bishop (1994, p. 36) have offered clear guidance for a focus of clinical supervision towards that of the management of professional practice in identifying aims of:

- Safeguarding standards of practice
- Development of professional expertise
- Delivery of quality care.

However, despite the management functions in many of the nursing models and approaches being described in essentially positive terms, with clear links to quality assurance, the monitoring of standards and promotion of clinical effectiveness, practitioners have remained suspicious of this component within clinical supervision (Jones, 1995; Wilkin *et al.* 1997). Negative interpretations remain as do anxieties that information shared could be used to discipline practitioners (Payne, 1999).

Given the apparent sensitivities within nursing and the negativity surrounding previous supervisory approaches, it may have been more productive to have avoided the negative associations of introducing a management aspect borrowed from other disciplines. It may also have been more beneficial to retain the purity of Proctor's earlier ideas, as that of a partnership, driven by self-valuing, self-assessing and enabling responsibilities. Proctor's formulations of formative, normative and restorative tasks have their own specific meaning that further suggest a more enabling relationship than that ascribed by some nursing authors. The shared tasks of supervision as identified by Proctor (1986) and Inskipp & Proctor (1993) are laid out in Table 4.1.

Within Proctor's framework, supervision is much more about the shared responsibilities within a supportive, as well as creative, working alliance that assists practitioners to move from the 'human doing' to the 'human

Table 4.1 The shared tasks of supervision.

Formative: (development)	developing skills and enhancing understanding, building on practitioner's abilities, enabling personal and professional development.
Normative: (assessment)	shared responsibilities for monitoring standards and the ethical practice of the practitioner, through self-assessment and valuing contributions.
Restorative: (refreshment and creativity)	relating to the affective or emotional domain, allowing for the sharing of feelings and discharging and recharging of emotions and energies.

being' ethos of the therapeutic approach. This may not be an easy transition to make given the current culture of the NHS, and nurses in particular may experience difficulties in finding a space and someone suitable to reflect with about clinical performance and personal development.

Such a flexible framework, however, does match well with the growth and development approaches sensitively explored and proposed by Faugier (1998). These types of relationships allow those in clinical practice to make the connections for their own development more readily, as separate from any managerial inference that may be considered overseeing or monitoring. Supervision so defined becomes a suitable enabling relationship for preparing individual practitioners in becoming self-directed and autonomous.

As one practitioner reports, clinical supervision should promote self-evaluation and self-worth, as well as evaluation of clinical and therapeutic interactions, to offer a validation of clinical practice and individual performance (P. Davies, 1993). Self-management is an integral part of the supervision process and is achieved within a supportive, restorative relationship that enables professional growth and development within the relative boundaries of the organisational culture.

Hawkins and Shohet (1989) reinforce this perspective and recommend supervision as playing an important part of taking care of oneself, remaining open to new learning and facilitating self-awareness and continued commitment to learning. These are essential elements of becoming an effective practitioner in one's own field and are part of the process that requires supervisory relationships to be built on the essential assumptions that practitioners in the service professions:

- Want to monitor their own performance
- Wish to learn to develop competence
- Will respond to support and encouragement (Proctor, 1986).

Proctor's work has been thoughtfully adapted and illustrated by Meg Bond and Stevie Holland (1998, p. 16), which goes some way towards exploring the various tasks or aspects of the original model, within the context of a nursing setting. Bond and Holland (1998) provide a comprehensive critical analysis, having drawn on their extensive experiences in working with supervisors and practitioners. This allows them to effectively inform and clarify the complexities of clinical supervision within the nursing context and offer a range of practical suggestions for carrying the initiative forward. These authors offer a fresh insight and acknowledge those who have assisted in the development of supervision from other professional and occupational fields, to inform nursing's notion of clinical supervision.

According to Bond and Holland (1998), the restorative and formative tasks of clinical supervision are the means by which the formative task is addressed in practice. However, the framework offered here develops the idea that all three tasks are involved in a delicate equilibrium for effective discharging and recharging of energies (support), developing (continuing professional development and education), and promoting individual competence (quality assurance and professional ethics).

This matches with what Hawkins and Shohet (1989) determine as the primary focus of supervision and by subtly shifting the balance, each of the restorative, educative and normative tasks can be dominant or recessive according to need, level of practice and particular context. As Hawkins and Shohet readily admit, there may be overlap and greater or lesser integration of tasks depending on the particular needs of the individual practitioner/supervisee and the context within which they practise.

In exploring the relationship of tasks and functions it is important to stress that the normative task is primarily concerned, in this case, with the development of individual competence through self-assessment and with personal performance review to promote individual responsibility and autonomy. Personal performance review is considered a personal and informal activity that facilitates the assessment of individual performance in everyday practice.

This is to be separated from the more formal individual performance review (IPR) or those appraisal systems which relate to management processes, with the assessment of performance relating to organisational roles, responsibilities, aims and outcomes. The two are of course compatible as self-assessment is a necessary part of IPR and appraisal, and the focus for this proposed framework rests on interpreting assessment and quality monitoring positively and providing a relationship where a pratitioner can be 'open and reflective about what he does know but can also acknowledge without loss of face what he does not know' (Westheimer, 1977, p. 19).

Building on and acknowledging the contributions of others demonstrates how Bond and Holland's (1998) work can be further adapted to continue the dialogue about this developing, professional support relationship. Figure 4.2 demonstrates the interlocking, enabling aspects or tasks of clinical supervision, set within the individual and cultural contexts. Having devised this framework I later discovered, when exploring further the literature on reflection, Fowler and Chevannes' (1998) interesting paper. They offer a similar perspective and diagrammatic representation to link reflection to clinical supervision.

The individual context relates to the particular needs of the practitioner and their level of practice or training requirements, recognising

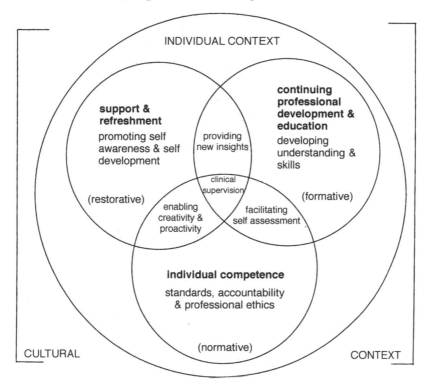

INDIVIDUAL CONTEXT

**support &
refreshment**
promoting self
awareness & self
development

providing
new insights

**continuing
professional
development &
education**
developing
understanding &
skills

clinical
supervision

(restorative)

enabling
creativity &
proactivity

facilitating
self assessment

(formative)

individual competence
standards, accountability
& professional ethics

CULTURAL

(normative)

CONTEXT

Figure 4.2:   The enabling functions of clinical supervision.

that clinical supervision should continue throughout professional life
(Butterworth, 1998). The cultural context which is integrally linked to
the organisational setting, identifies the professional tribe or occupational group, with both contexts instrumental in informing the category
of supervision to be selected. In nursing's case this is likely to be clinical
supervision, as independent supervision for registered practitioners and
tutorial and training supervision for the students engaged in pre-
registration education. The particular needs of students will be
discussed later in this chapter in relation to the roles available and how
they may develop in future.

The proposed framework for clinical supervision suggested here
attempts to remain true to the essence of Proctor's original deliberations
and this is reflected in making connections with the terminology used,
with the normative task being modified to relate to the newly emerging
quality initiatives in the NHS (DoH, 1998). However, as identified earlier,
this task should relate primarily to the competence of the individual,
allowing the practitioner to explore professional ethics, self-assessment
and individual standards of performance.

This informs our current working definition of clinical supervision as the debate continues, which is that of an interactive professional partnership where there is shared responsibility for stimulating critical reflection reviewing and assessing personal performance, as well as providing support and emotional refreshment.

Clinical governance presents a major shift in quality policy and draws together the differing quality assurance mechanisms in an attempt to improve clinical standards at local service levels and throughout the whole of the health service. This provides a comprehensive infrastructure involving competent leadership and accountability to mesh the various quality processes together. Known as clinical governance the intentions are to ensure responsibility and accountability through evidence-based guidelines developed by the National Institute of Clinical Effectiveness, set up in April 1999.

It is recognised that this initiative will have to be set within a broader framework of strategies for managing risk, providing for effective continuing professional development and the dissemination of good practice (Muir Gray, 1997; Gulland, 1999). With the development of such initiatives it becomes highly probable that professional support roles will have a vital part to play in supporting and developing practitioners. This has particular relevance for clinical supervision as one of the aims of clinical governance is that of establishing:

> 'the need to focus on the activities involved in delivering high quality care. It will mean the *creation of a systematic set of mechanisms that will support staff* and develop all health organisations to deliver a new approach to quality.'
>
> (NHS Executive, 1998, p. 2) [italics added]

The aims of clinical governance are encapsulated within a proposed vision for the following five years which identifies the following areas of change:

- A new culture in NHS organisations
- Addressing inequity and variability
- Involving users and carers
- The sharing of good practice
- Detecting and dealing with poor performance.

Within the overall vision there is recognition for the guidance on quality to be developmental and not prescriptive and this suggests a positive remit for quality monitoring to safeguard standards of care. It is therefore essential that the open and enabling style of this policy imperative is matched by clinical supervision processes that are creatively developed and sensitively implemented.

Making clinical supervision work in practice

Frameworks, models and definitions are helpful in illuminating clinical supervision but perhaps most important is that practitioners themselves engage in the debate and decide what they want clinical supervision to be and how it should evolve in practice. Certainly it is our view that for successful relationships to be developed there is a need for locally modified approaches, adapted to the local context and policy requirements and individual practitioner's needs, and taking into account the effects on patient/client care (Wolsey & Leach, 1997; Wright *et al.*, 1997).

We appreciate the helpful discussions of Hawkins and Shohet (1989) in setting the scene for deliberations that ensure that clinical supervision is open and enabling, with supervision providing a safe space for reflection in and on practice. This would appear to go some way towards modifying the negative perceptions for as Christopher Maggs reminds us, we need to consider carefully how we approach clinical supervision in order to prevent 'another instance of professional regression' (Maggs, 1998, p. 41).

For clinical supervision to be a success and for it to become embedded within the culture of nursing and health care, particularly at the cutting edge of care delivery, it is essential that this professional support relationship is placed in context with the others that are available (as will be explored in Chapter 5) and with the other practice and educational initiatives such as the introduction of reflection, portfolio development and continuing professional education requirements. There is also a need to emphasise such initiatives within the context of the need for continuing learning and critical challenge in practice.

If clinical supervision is to be owned, developed and implemented appropriately, then it is essential for those busy practitioners who would best benefit from this type of relationship to come to an understanding of what they want from clinical supervision and how it would work best in practice. This shifts the rather passive, didactic questions of what it is and how to do it, to what do we want from clinical supervision and how will we achieve this? The balance of responsibility and ownership for the initiative passes to the very practitioners who can make it a worthwhile experience that benefits both themselves and others. If clinical supervision is truly a partnership, then educators and researchers should collaborate with practitioners and managers in a spirit of creativity and innovation to develop effective enabling frameworks (Morton-Cooper & Bamford, 1997). As Dolan (1998, p. 5) recommends, there should be a 'shared understanding that there is no one way to do it'.

In the recent past emphasis has been placed on extolling the benefits of clinical supervision, which have been stressed by a range of sources. However, the empirical evidence is scarce and inconclusive and there remains work to do (Wolsey & Leach, 1997; Butterworth *et al.*, 1998). Such benefits that are readily shared and highlighted include improved patient care through reflective practice; dissemination of good practice; shared learning; support for continuing professional development encouraging a sharing culture; exchange of ideas; increased job satisfaction; improved patient/client care; reduced staff turnover and increased motivation. There is a real danger that clinical supervision could be seen by some as a panacea for a multitude of deficiencies in professional and organisational systems.

Despite the emerging and sometimes ambivalent evidence there is clearly a need for further empirical endeavours to identify the benefits and rewards of clinical supervision in practice, as well as attempts to discover and measure its impact on patient/client care (Wilson-Barnett *et al.*, 1995; Butterworth *et al.*, 1996; Norman, 1998). Extravagant claims were made in the early deliberations of the possible benefits. However, as many authors identify, there is a real need for appropriate evaluation. The key question is not whether clinical supervision will have a positive outcome, but more importantly how clinical supervision will affect the quality of the service delivered. Such explorations should also include how it will assist in developing and equipping practitioners for the future.

From working within a series of acute and community health care trusts, using a variety of evaluative approaches including focus groups and nominal group techniques, staff identified a list of benefits and outcomes during the implementation of clinical supervision (Wilson & Palmer, 1999). These are shown in Table 4.2. However, once again it is

Table 4.2 Outcomes and benefits of clinical supervision.

Encourages sharing of ideas between practitioners and enhances patient care
Facilitates better team working
Encourages reflection on practice
Allows exploration of alternative approaches to care
Promotes better communication
Provides a more focused service to patients
Increases professional support
Helps increase practitioner's confidence
Helps combat stress

---

important to stress that individual supervisors and practitioners must discover the benefits for themselves as they take responsibility for how clinical supervision shapes up in their particular context. These benefits also have to be considered in relation to the barriers to clinical supervision that are emerging – insufficient time, pressure of work, shortage of staff and difficulties in coordinating the process. This supports the findings of others and unless these areas are addressed, there is a real risk that they will eventually derail the clinical supervision bandwagon, (Marrow *et al.*, 1997; Wilson & Palmer, 1999).

If clinical supervision is to be successfully integrated into the culture of nursing by busy practitioners, it must be recognised that this is a relationship that can be instrumental and significant in:

- Benefiting both practitioners and patients/clients
- Promoting lifelong learning
- Developing an enabling culture of health care built on openness and trust
- Playing its part in the span of supportive frameworks.

For this recognition to gain credence and be appreciated by those it would best benefit we have also found that there is a need for:

- Clear policy guidelines
- Support from management and identified product champions
- Clarity of communication and connection with other Trust and NHS initiatives
- Sound leadership
- Effective resource provision.

It is all very well to suggest that practitioners should take on board clinical supervision, but they require time to reflect and mull over their current work patterns and identify how such relationships can work for them in their world of work. This is essential if they are to take on board and prevent clinical supervision from becoming yet another misplaced nursing innovation (Salvage, 1998).

In recommending a critical questioning and a reflective approach, John's model of professional supervision (John, 1993) gives direction on how to alter the balance towards practitioners' needs, helping them to to make sense of themselves, their world of work and the supportive relationships they require. In encouraging contemplation about any method of professional support and in this case clinical supervision, it is useful for practitioners to begin with the practicalities by asking themselves:

- How has my work/role changed in recent years?
- What are the increasing demands and how do I cope with them?
- How am I maintaining my continuing professional education?
- What do I do to ensure that I learn in practice and from my experiences?

These are relevant questions that begin the process of thinking and reflecting on work situations and relationships, encouraging individual practitioners to engage with their own needs. They are questions that move the individual from the more easily recognisable and somewhat passive learning, with pragmatic questions: Are you coping? Do you want support for professional development? are you experiencing difficulties in delivering quality care and do you need help? This last question may be particularly difficult to own up to in a professional culture that has traditionally not placed a major emphasis on 'caring for the carers'.

It should be acknowledged that encouraging practitioners to take a more reflective approach in making decisions about their own needs for development and support may well open up important issues for them. For those nurses wishing to develop more assertive approaches (McCoppin & Gardener, 1994) and get to grips with marketing their unique talents (Hudson-Jones, 1988), there are broader questions that link this relationship to the quality remit:

- How do I know what I am doing?
- How do I know that I am doing it well?
- How can I value what I do?
- How can I maintain my creativity?

These are the very issues that can be explored within a clinically focused relationship that provides a space for reflection, guidance, informal performance review and professional support. There is a need to identify what we mean by taking a 'reflective approach', as there is more to reflection than an 'educational buzz-word' which reduces it to keeping a diary. Reflection concerns active processes and strategies that involve the maintenance of learning records in the form of profiles or portfolios (Johns, 1993; Palmer, 1997). Some educators, perhaps in their enthusiasm for engaging with the works of Schon (1983) and Boud *at al.*, (1985) have not been able to easily transfer this enthusiasm to those working in practice (McCormack & Hopkins, 1995; Brady, 1998).

Learning in practice and clinical supervision

We believe reflection and related activities such as critical thinking and adult learning are integral to learning in practice and to the whole notion of making clinical supervision a practical reality.

There is increasing recognition for learning in practice, in the work-place and from our personal and professional experiences, as we make sense of the world around us and take on new meanings (Bines & Watson, 1992; Miller & Boud, 1996). There is also recognition for the learning that arises from both formal (education programmes and study days) and informal learning (our experience, on the wards and in practice). Most practitioners will recognise certain situations or events that appear to change their thinking, resulting in a change of behaviour, attitude or feelings.

Learning from experience or experiential learning involves engaging with cycles of inquiry which lead to experimentation, with the trying out and testing of new ideas and actions in practice. Experiential learning also allows the drawing together of fragments of experience and encourages 'ways of knowing' by working with, and interpreting, the patterns and connections of real life experiences (Weil & McGill, 1989). This involves reflective processes and approaches that were first proposed by educational theorists and teachers many years ago, in attempting to make sense of how individuals learn in everyday life and work situations (Dewey, 1938; Freire, 1972; Kolb, 1984).

Effective connections for the professional world and the nature of professional knowledge and knowing in action have been made by Benner (1984), Barnett (1992) and Eraut (1994), and reflection has increasingly become an important component in encouraging practitioners to explore and learn from their world of practice (Cox, 1992).

Reflection – capturing experience

The notion of capturing experience and mulling it over, leading to new insights and new actions, is what reflection is all about (Boud *et al.*, 1985). It is an important part of learning that brings meaning to practice, and despite now being relatively well documented in nursing (Atkins & Murphy, 1993; Palmer *et al.*, 1994), it remains a somewhat difficult and illusive concept to grasp (James & Clarke, 1994; Tsang, 1998) and with limited evidence of the 'how to do' elements (Driscoll, 2000). It is notable that in the past many reflective activities have centred on the keeping of diaries and learning journals, to the detriment of the thinking processes and support structures that can facilitate reflection in practice (Carr, 1996).

Donald Schon was one of the first to excite the nursing education world with his interpretations of reflection, involving both reflection-on-action, the retrospective activities, and reflection-in-action, the reflexive activities as in exploring 'the here and now' (Schon, 1983). This offered clarity for some, while others initially appeared slightly less enamoured with the approach (Eraut, 1994). Interestingly, in nursing as Gary Rolfe notes, the literature has tended to focus on reflection-on-action activities and less on reflection-in-action activities, which also have relevance to learning in practice (Rolfe, 1998).

There appears to be general agreement in nursing and the other health professions that reflection assists learning from experience in helping practitioners to think about what they do, to understand what they do, and most importantly to analyse experiences (Horton, 1990). There is also some consensus that sound examples are required from practice to give a personal perspective and get to grips with the issues and challenges of what it means to be a reflective practitioner. There are those who offer such insights and living examples of what engaging in reflection means in reality, and the issues, challenges and practicalities that have to be addressed (L'Aiguille, 1994; Johns & Graham, 1996; Routledge *et al.*, 1997; Jasper, 1998). Reflection offers new dimensions and this is beautifully encapsulated by L'Aiguille (1994, pp. 86–7) who records that 'reflecting in action has increased my ability to look upon my world with eyes other than my own'.

In considering the connections between learning in practice and reflection, it is sensible to explore how experiential learning and the fruitful analysis of experience are informed by the other learning approaches that engender reflective practice. These approaches and strategies have been developed from the initial, experiential studies and concern adult learning and critical thinking or critical reasoning (Knowles, 1984; Brookfield, 1987; Argyris, 1991).

In adult learning the responsibility and motivation for learning is firmly placed with the individual, who by applying problem solving abilities and critical thinking is self-directed and takes responsibility for his/her learning (Knowles, 1984). Adult learning with its emphasis on process not content confirms learning as an active process with adult learners seeking their own paths of discovery – in analysing, evaluating and fully experiencing their world of work.

Critical thinking is an important component of adult learning as it relates to abilities to challenge the assumptions that formulate our ideas, actions, values and beliefs and makes us attempt alternative ways of thinking and acting (Brookfield, 1987). As a result of such deliberations, the effective professional is expected to be continuously self-critical, but it must be acknowledged and recognised by both educators and practitioners that there is 'no single right way for thinking critically' (Wallace 1996, p. 47) and that historically 'contemporary nursing is dogged by a negative expectation that nurses should not think' (Dartington, 1994, p. 101).

How do individuals become critical thinkers? The responsibility may well lie with the balance between the individual practitioner engaging in a critical dialogue with themselves (in what Hawkins and Shohet (1987) have determined as self-supervision) and having a critical discourse with another (a mentor or clinical supervisor). Developing critical thinking skills also involves the application of a reflective approach that is founded on the sound use of observational skills, active listening and analytical reading as well as the sharing of ideas (van den Brink-Budgen, 1996; Clarke & Croft, 1998). There is further evidence that being part of an organisational climate that is proactive in encouraging continual learning and innovation, and encourages support in practice, is highly beneficial (Sadler, 1989; Swierings & Wierdsma, 1992).

Such approaches fit well with the principles of a learning organisation whereby individuals are expected to continually challenge and develop new ideas as well as question what they and others are doing, within an environment of openness and trust. It is also important in developing critical thinking that significant experiences, both positive and negative, are captured and worked on and for some this process has become known as portfolio-based learning (James, 1990; Simosko, 1991).

Portfolio-based learning – a personal, reflective guide

Portfolio-based learning is steadily gaining impetus in nursing, medical and social work education, with developing interest from the other health care therapies (Pietroni & Millard, 1996; GLPQ, 1997; Routledge *et al.*, 1997.) Portfolio-based learning is much more than making brief notes now and again in a journal or reflective diary, or even writing up six weeks experiences the night before it is due to be handed in as course work. It is a personal record of individual abilities and motivations that encourages further learning from experience.

A portfolio is a structured record of achievement which contains an analysis and record of learning experiences and forms an integral part of the reflection process and the development of critical thinking (McGrowther, 1995; Pietroni & Palmer, 1995; Teasdale, 1996). There is some confusion in British nursing between portfolios and profiles, which has not been helped by the differing interpretations offered by some of the statutory and regulatory bodies (ENB, 1994; UKCC, 1995).

A commonly understood comparison of what they are and what they contain is given by Ros Brown. The profile provides particular infor-

mation for a specified purpose and identified audience, while the portfolio is a comprehensive record of learning events (both formal and
informal), incidents, feelings, achievements and curriculum vitae – in
fact any item, thought or comment that assists learning and makes you
think about experiences and practice (Brown, 1995).

The portfolio is a live document that is your own critical safe space
where you can record what you like and reflect on it at leisure. It is a
collection of your notes, reading, handouts, learning opportunities,
activities you have completed, documents you have collected, and most
importantly, your reflections about your work or practice. Effective
portfolio learning means that you have to work with the entries in a
meaningful and reflective way by posing questions and challenging the
assumptions that you make about events and learning situations
(Mitchell & Shaw, 1994; Hull & Redfern, 1996).

There are those who support the idea of identifying and using critical
incidents to assist the reflective process, and this is useful advice
(Crouch, 1991; Rich & Parker, 1995), but it is also important to work
regularly with your thoughts, emotions and reflections and update your
records accordingly. As Williams (1998, p. 30) comments, 'the focus of
learning is upon critical analysis of that unique practice situation'. It is
also important to remember that this is a dynamic document that supports learning from experience; it will help in the questioning of
assumptions and will allow you to make connections and comparisons
with similar situations and events (Jasper, 1998). Recording your
experiences in this way helps you plan for further learning and this can
be achieved by completing a personal action plan to include in your
portfolio. An example of a plan is given in Table 4.3.

It is vital to appreciate that it is not just writing in your portfolio that is
important, but it is the continuing critical analysis and reflection on what
has been written that assists you in benefiting and learning from your
experiences. This critical analysis involves reviewing an event, identifying what you already know, challenging assumptions and creatively
exploring alternatives (Burnard, 1989; Clarke & Croft, 1998). The following points are offered as guidance when working with your portfolio
entries and are based on the reflections of Pietroni & Palmer (1994).

Working with your portfolio

The portfolio is a personal document and there is no right or wrong way
to maintain it. You may be asked to provide information from it (the
personal professional profile – UKCC, 1995) for accreditation of practice, but the reflective elements and working with your experiences can,
and should, remain private and personal.

Table 4.3   Clinical Supervision – A personal action plan.

You can analyse and value what you are learning by:
- Identifying the clinical, managerial or organisational issues that you bring to the clinical supervision sessions.
- Reflecting on what you have explored in each session.
- Examining your current practice in relation to the areas/situations covered.
- Identifying and sharing any further learning needs.
- Making decisions about how and where the new learning can be used.

Action taken

You can devise a plan for putting learning into practice by:
- Planning what you want to achieve.
- Identifying the areas of practice you want to develop.
- Setting realistic aims and time for completion.
- Identifying relevant resources and further learning support.
- Reviewing and evaluating your progress with your clinical supervisor.

Action taken

You can record what you have achieved by:
- Reporting your reflections to these activities and recording other learning opportunities that happen.
- Maintaining a personal record of the progress that you are making.
- Writing a critical review showing how you have changed or adapted your practice.

Action taken

Source: (Palmer, 1992)

It is important to seek out the method of working with your notes that best suits you as it is essential that the entries concern you and your learning experiences. You can be frank and honest about what you think and feel as the most important aspect is to be yourself.

Be confident in working with and shaping the portfolio; engage with it regularly and allow your thoughts to flow freely. It is much easier to write and then stand back and reflect on what you have written.

Use diagrams, pictures, newspaper cuttings or other types of material to record feelings and responses to particular situations. A symbol, illustration or cartoon can express an idea or emotion very effectively.

The portfolio forms a learning work-book and entries that demonstrate relevant connections and new insights should be highlighted. Such activities will engage you with your thoughts and feelings as well as encourage learning.

Be spontaneous and say what you feel, ask yourself critical questions, record your deliberations, work with them and respond to issues that surface as you reflect.

Keeping a portfolio is an important part of learning in practice and from experience but it it is also important to acknowledge the other strategies and learning activities that complement these personal reflections.

Seeing the patterns – completing the jigsaw

For learning in practice and reflection to become fundamental facets of practice there is a need to recognise that there should be effective organisational measures, as well as an identified vehicle for the activities and processes that facilitate reflective practice. Organisational measures and structures involve the provision of an effective learning ethos or learning organisation culture that involves appropriate continuing professional development strategies, effective resource identification and firm management commitment for integrating such approaches into the working day.

An effective vehicle for reflection may well be that of clinical supervision, which has been identified as having a significant role in providing a suitable relationship for analysing and developing practice (Fisher, 1996; UKCC, 1996). Other authors have brought together the processes of action research and critical reflection (Weil, 1998) whereas in nursing links have been made between action research, clinical supervision and reflective practice (Graham, 1995; Moore & Carter, 1998). Fish & Twinn (1997) identify strands of reflection to provide a focus for the analysis of practice, which involves personal narratives, retrospective reviews, exploring assumptions and making the relevant connections to inform future practice.

In this discussion the connections are made between relevant learning approaches and strategies, reflective practice and clinical supervision. The skills, functions and tasks applicable to clinical supervision can be demonstrated in the interactions between the inquiry approaches of experiential learning, adult learning, critical thinking and portfolio-based learning. These are brought together with the processes of reviewing, reflecting and recording, processes that were developed and proved instrumental in assisting role transition and encouraging learning from practice, within the innovative *Nursing Times* open learning programme (Palmer, 1993).

The approaches and processes are then set within the context of practice and are influenced by the practice setting or organisational context. The context will change according to the professional status and learning needs of the individual practitioner. For example, for clinical practitioners the context will be clinical/professional and for managers it will be managerial/professional, while for students it will be the education/clinical/professional who is required to engage with the range of interconnecting approaches, in a continual cycle of 'learning to learn' from experience. (See Fig. 4.3.)

In asking, and in some cases expecting, practitioners to become reflective practitioners, it should be appreciated that working with

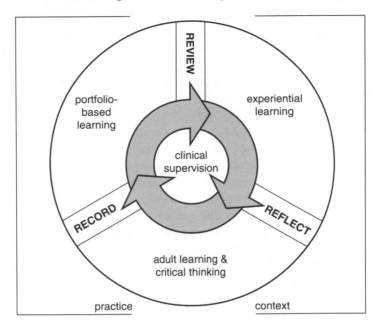

Fig. 4.3   Learning approaches and strategies involved in clinical supervision.

portfolio entries, analysing practice, critically examining roles and learning to reflect may lead to the release of strong emotions, even defensive reactions (Argyris, 1991; Wallace, 1996). Reflection can be accompanied by an awareness of uncomfortable feelings, and exploring difficult situations can produce negative feelings that may be a barrier to learning (Boud, *et al.*, 1985; Boud & Walker, 1996).

If clinical supervision is truly a supportive relationship that provides a focus for shared learning, developing and restoring self, and identifying learning needs, then it has a role to play in supporting reflective practice; and if clinical supervision is seen as the formal system, then reflection appears to be its enabling process (Fowler & Chevannes, 1998, p. 380). Whilst their initial research findings indicate that there is a high degree of compatibility between reflective practice and clinical supervision, Fowler & Chevannes draw our attention to the view that reflection should not always be seen as an integral part of clinical supervision. It is suggested that such an approach may be avoided by practitioners, unused and unable to cope with reflective activities.

This is a sound supposition and one that has to be taken on board by those of us who consider reflective practice to be an important part of learning in practice (Johns, 1993; UKCC, 1996; Palmer, 1997). If reflection is to play a part in clinical supervision this will have significant implications for the preparation of both supervisors and practitioners, with clear understanding of the process of clinical supervision and all those involved having experienced clinical supervision (Cutcliffe & Proctor, 1998).

As the concept of clinical supervision is explored it becomes increasingly obvious that it has a significant part to play within the repertoire of professional support roles. Having discussed the origins and interpretations and how it may appear in clinical practice, it seems sensible to identify how such a relationship may be adapted for those starting out in their chosen careers and occupations, before concluding with the common questions that are raised by the practitioners who work with and shape the student experience.

The student as a new arrival has specific educational, clinical learning and support needs and the following discussions will highlight some familiar support roles as well as introduce different, modified roles in the form of a broader interpretation for meeting the needs of the group of fledgling practitioners.

Supervision and support for the student

Student support is complemented by a wider network of significant others in the form of their peers, and educational advisers who may be designated as personal tutors or academic advisers. Such roles are identified in relation to student needs, but it is worth noting that any qualified practitioner who registers for a further course of study will have access to this form of support and guidance. In considering the particular needs for students, the roles of tutorial and training supervision appear as sensible options and this will be explored through the identification of the specific coaching functions suitable for a professional support relationship of this type.

It is our view that clinical supervision should commence at the point of entry to the profession, as an ensuring–enabling relationship is vital as the student adjusts and aclimatises to the professional practice environment. This is perhaps more obvious now that the limitations of Project 2000 have been revealed and a practice skills deficiency identified in those registered and ready to practice (Jowett, *et al.*, 1994; Maben & Macleod Clark, 1997).

Peers and peer groups

A peer is a colleague who is of similar status within the organisation, someone who forms a collaborative relationship that is often mutually rewarding. The relationship is also non-competitive as the group of peers forms an informal and supportive social network where the individuals relate together as colleagues and friends.

As discussed earlier in the chapter, health care is becoming more complicated, change more rapid and demands for care provision more exacting. Similar demands are now occurring in professional and higher education, and changes in the student population, with the numbers of mature students gradually increasing and living patterns changing, have meant fewer opportunities for the formal and informal exchanges of previous education programmes. These were characterised by the shared practices that arose from close working relationships in clinical placements, and by informal opportunities to reflect on practical experiences arising from living in communal establishments within close proximity to the patients (Northcott, 1998b)

Peers and peer groups can provide the student with a close, social network that can be very beneficial, allowing the student to gain a great deal from this type of liaison. Remaining as part of the group can assist the student in checking his/her personal progress within the relative safety of a group of colleagues of similar standing. The desire to make use of the potential benefits of this sort of grouping has led to the setting up of more formal systems of peer groups: peer tutorials, the Open University self help groups, the *Nursing Times* open learning student study groups and the 'buddy' systems of North America. All these systems offer a variety of approaches to help students become part of their own independently directed learning groups, and this leads to increasing initiatives for student contributions to peer review, peer audit, peer tutoring, peer mentoring, peer evaluation and informal co-counselling techniques (Mockford, 1994; Topping, 1994; Yates *et al.*, 1997).

The roles and responsibilities of academic advisers

Academic advisers have a central role to play in supporting students through an education programme, being assigned to students to assist with their progress while they are on the course. They do this by helping the student to set his/her own realistic academic goals or targets which can then be worked towards. The student is encouraged to be self-directed and to make the most of the learning opportunities that occur during and outside the time-tabled sessions of the curriculum.

The academic adviser is usually a member of the course team and this knowledge of the course programme and commitments eases the student through the rigours of academic life. This has become an increasingly important priority as new educational initiatives are placed on the educational agenda. Initiatives of accreditation of prior learning

and accreditation of prior experiential learning have resulted in increasing numbers of mature students with different abilities. This is providing educational managers, lecturers and advisors with the challenges of managing the increasing numbers and discovering new methods and approaches of encouraging learning (Ramsden, 1992; Hull & Redfern, 1996).

Choosing the right course and working through modules, as well as pressures of continuing assessment and self-direction, make it appropriate for the student to have a significant academic helper. Changing social circumstances and taking increasing responsibility for their own learning and progression through a course may increase risks of student isolation. Students are obliged to know who to contact in order to ensure that their academic needs will be met (Rickards, 1992). The responsibility for arranging meetings and tutorials rests with the student, who is encouraged to meet regularly in order for the academic adviser to assist in assessing their progress and helping them to reach their full academic potential. The specific roles and functions of the academic adviser are listed below and demonstrate the range of responsibilities that play a major part in the student's academic development. The links between this type of relationship and that of tutorial supervision are clearly evident.

For the individual student, the responsibilities of the academic adviser are (University of London, 1992):

To help:
- Make the most effective use of time
- Plan an individual programme of work
- Set realistic targets
- Choose the options that best meet personal needs, interests and career plans
- Liaise with the teaching staff or registry.

To reflect:
- On individual development in relation to the course, and to chart progress.

To monitor:
- Progress on the course in light of the personal and academic goals set.

To provide:
- Advice and career references that may be required in the future.

In this manner the student is given support that reflects his/her individual learning needs during a course of study. The academic support and assistance relates to all aspects of the course, including help with organisational aspects such as administration, and extends beyond the end of the course to the working world.

Personal tutors

Another common support role with similar responsibilities to the academic adviser is the personal tutor. As a member of the teaching staff the personal tutor is important, providing the student with support and having 'responsibilities for keeping a watchful eye on the student's work and progress on an individual basis' (Earwaker, 1992, pp. 45–6).

Traditionally in nursing education, medicine and other health care programmes, the personal tutor has had responsibilities that extend beyond those of the academic adviser (Taylor, 1980). As well as assisting with the student's academic progress the personal tutor had responsibilities for pastoral care and for overseeing the student's progress through practice placements, a remit which appears to fit well with tutorial supervision activities as identified earlier in this chapter in the discussion on decoding supervision. Prior to the Project 2000 courses and the change of student status to that of supernumary, the personal tutor's counselling role did not always fit easily with the management responsibilities of 'the employed student'. Recognising this, counselling services were developed in some nursing schools, but in the main, student counselling responsibilities remained with the personal tutor.

In higher education, pastoral support is available from a variety of institutional sources such as student services and specialised telephone help-lines. The academic adviser can therefore concentrate on helping the student with his/her academic needs and can assist with appropriate counselling referrals should the need arise. The clear distinction in responsibilities is made and the personal tutor's role is to assist the student to set their own learning agenda 'within a business-like working relationship' (Earwaker, 1992).

Setting the scene – supervision and facilitation

A variety of key roles have previously been identified in providing learning support for students in clinical placements and these have been instrumental in developing those new to the professional working world. In social work and occupational therapy, clinical supervisors have traditionally had responsibilities for assisting learning and clinical socialisation. In midwifery, health visiting and nursing, the roles of clinical supervisors, field work practice teachers, clinical teachers, assessors and latterly mentors have been established to enhance learning and provide learning support. The emphasis in the past has been on the use of clinical teaching to prepare students and provide role models for practice.

Facilitation

Facilitation appears to have been a more acceptable term to some practitioners who remained sceptical about the enabling tasks of supervision and the role it could play in helping them focus on practice. Hopefully with the current debate and emerging approaches that do not carry the negative connotations of history, supervision will be accepted and will find its rightful place in professional support frameworks. The art of facilitation has been well documented in the health care professions; for example, its involvement in personal development, developing interpersonal skills and assisting with the affective domains, widely used since the early deliberations of educationalists and psychologists (Rogers, 1969; Heron, 1977). Facilitation now forms an important part of the learning process and is effective in providing a non-directive, non-confrontational, flexible environment to assist student learning and development (Cameron, 1998; Heron, 1999).

In practice the facilitator acts as a learning resource, creating the necessary climate for learning and offering guidance as required. Proficient facilitators are experienced and have patience to allow their students to be self-directed, but are able to appreciate when their interventions are requested or needed. To promote effective learning, facilitative relationships have to be based on trust, respect and a genuine valuing of each other's abilities. It is clear that such a role fits well with the current ethos of adult learning, and with the introduction of co-facilitation techniques the scene is set for developing effective collaborative partnerships (Knight & Scott, 1998).

General nursing, in particular, having experienced difficulties with the less positive elements of the supervisor's role, with the emphasis on monitoring, admonishing and negative feedback, has tended to see facilitation as a positive alternative. Certainly it would appear sensible to consider roles that combine the enabling aspects of facilitation with the practicalities of coaching functions, and this is perhaps where training and tutorial supervision have a part to play. This could form the basis of a new direction for so called 'clinical supervisory' learning support, and by adding specific coaching functions could extend its meaning for more general use. It could also aid its acceptability, as adult learning approaches and developing professional accountability continue to influence the practice domain.

Coaching

'Coaching' is a relatively new term and it is one that may not rest easily in British health culture and nursing service. We believe it could be developed and used to balance the negative impressions that still surround the notion of 'supervision' despite the addition of the prefix 'clinical'.

Coaching is a prerequisite for allowing students to develop effective skills and abilities within a supportive exchange of instruction, advice and positive feedback. The term coaching in education has been borrowed from the sporting world and is commonly found in commercial organisations where the emphasis is on productivity and competition and where coaching relates to activities of team effort and achievement (Kelly, 1992). Extending this role beyond that applied in sport and business makes it necessary to adapt and clarify the functional elements of coaching – such as monitoring, assessment, instruction and feedback, – in a manner that it is conducive to a student entering a professional field of study and practice. Here the emphasis is on giving service and caring and a broader interpretation of coaching would place value on the humanistic theories of learning and vocational influences.

We consider coaching involves helping individuals to improve their performance, to develop their skills and self confidence and to take on greater responsibility. Parsloe (1995) considers that mentoring and coaching are similar but distinct activities where the distinction for providing the appropriate type of support has to be clear. Parsloe also makes a comparison by exploring the origins of both roles – mentoring in advising and counselling, coaching in the immediate improvement of performance and development of practical skills by tutoring and instructing.

There are those who consider coaching as a means of improving performance for those that are already relatively proficient, rather than establishing competency (Weightman, 1996). This perspective does appear to fit with the coaching role as contemplated with the core assisting relationships of classical mentoring in what Tomlinson (1995) refers to as the 'reflective coach'. However, others do not see it this way and view it as a role that assists those in training to perform at their best, where strengths and weaknesses can be explored and opportunities are provided for relearning (Carter, 1993; Atherton, 1999):

> 'The most critical components of the coach role will be the capacity to demonstrate skills, communicate knowledge, and demonstrate appropriate attitudes within a well planned performance review and improvement strategy.'

> (Carter, 1993, p. 146)

Although probably aimed at the business workplace, such components resonate within professional practice and may well fit the developing lecturer–practitioner or staff nurse–student relationship, now that the demise of the clinical teacher role is complete.

Coaching then is perhaps a more acceptable concept for the new millennium as a collaborative ethos unfolds and new structures and differing relationships develop. The modification to include and stress coaching functions, has been made primarily to offset the negative images of clinical supervision as a support relationship with author-itarian overtones (Hill, 1989). Once the enabling and ensuring aspects are readily shared and clearly explained, and when both students and those they work with in practice are engaging in some form of clinical supervision, this type of relationship will gain the recognition and appreciation that it deserves.

The concern that clinical supervision remains unacceptable tells us more about the nature of nursing than it does about the nature of supervision as a mechanism for developing and supporting students.

Clinical supervision for students

In appreciating that clinical supervision is a delicate relationship that necessitates a sensitive balance of enabling and ensuring functions, it would appear to fit the needs of students in any proposed professional support framework. Clinical supervision as coaching supervision, applied appropriately, could be instrumental in encouraging new ways of establishing student support in the practice setting and emphasising the attainment of practical skills, self-assessment and evaluation by others. The clinical supervision relationship for students, it is suggested, should draw on the two complementary roles, with facilitation providing the enabling aspect of the relationship, while coaching promotes the ensuring functions that frame the professional standards and ethical expectations. It is envisaged that both aspects should work in harmony to enhance student learning and clinical development in practice placements.

This adaptation of 'training supervision', as it appears in the therapy domains, may appear contentious at this time of misused labels and confusion in roles. It has, however, been chosen in an attempt to broaden the functions and responsibilities of the training-supervisor role and to highlight the interactive, interpersonal processes that involve the acquisition of appropriate skills, actions and abilities that form the basis of professional practice. We see the role of the clinical supervisor as supervisor–coach for students, as instrumental in providing support for the new arrival to the profession and in meeting his/her specific learning needs.

Training supervision – roles and responsibilities of the supervisor–coach

Training supervision with a focus on coaching can facilitate constructive monitoring and positive feedback of performance to help the student make sense of the professional world they are entering. Allowing students to set their own learning agendas, within flexible parameters of guidance and assistance, will encourage self-awareness and ensure they take responsibility for their own learning needs, which, in turn, are compatible with the standards expected.

This type of supportive relationship fits well with the notion of creating reflective practitioners and Schon's (1988), view of developing professional and critical reflection is helping to adjust the balances between theory and practice. Indeed, as was noted earlier, it was Schon's work that raised the current interest in coaching and began the search to legitimise the use of the term in preparing new students for their professional, working world. He used it to provide the guide to his 'virtual world', setting educators on the quest of identifying the knowledge that underpins professional performance and informs on, in and during practice.

Based on these interpretations a supervisor–coach assists students to understand the nature of their role in professional practice and provides learning opportunities that allow the student to perform effectively. The supervisor–coach functions by negotiating and setting the ground rules, and offering guidance as well as instructions to the individual or team. This promotes discussion, constructive feedback and analysis for those involved as well as facilitating refinement of further practical effort carried out by the individual or team.

The coaching supervision process involves working through problems, setting appropriate outcomes and carrying out mutually agreed actions, followed by recognition of what has been achieved by all those involved (Fournies, 1978; Dale, 1998). Offering positive, constructive feedback enhances the student's experiences because it is individual and unique to the student's requirements and it can allow the free exchange of ideas based on observations and the mutually agreed outcomes. The focus of the activity remains the needs of the student and the analysis and feedback on his/her performance to encourage further learning, (Spouse, 1996).

The advice and counsel that follow allow discussion of a particular situation or set of events, providing a clear workable example that the student can focus on and explore to formulate differing ways of behaving. This implies a close working relationship between supervisor–coach and the student. It also provides a setting for critical reflection and fits well with problem solving approaches and experiential learning techniques. If used well and sensitively tuned to the student's needs, this facet of 'partnership in care' could go some way towards bridging the theory practice divide. It should also form one of the components of a constructive plan for assisting the student to reflect in and on practice.

Checklist of key functions of the supervisor–coach

A supervisor–coach can assist in the development of skills and behaviours for effective professional practice by utilising a balance of core and specific enabling characteristics.

Core enabling characteristics:
- Motivating students to set their own agenda for learning
- Providing safe opportunities for critical reflection
- Advising, counselling and guiding
- Assisting students to learn through their successes and failures
- Being an effective role model
- Recognising and supporting the student's strengths
- Developing the student's capabilities by offering constructive feedback.

Specific enabling characteristics:
- Assisting with student's progress in the practice placements
- Assisting the student to explore their practice
- Assessing and evaluating the student's performance
- Teaching, instructing and facilitating skills development
- Creating an environment of 'loving challenge'.

The supervisor–coach can set appropriate standards but it is the students themselves who work at them and by the 'doing' are gaining the experience that can be reflected on for future practice. In this manner students add to their repertoire of knowledge, experience and skills and begin their entry to the profession.

It is certainly time to address the confusing state of affairs concerning professional support, and those in service and education can collaborate in examining the range of support options available and can set the scene in order for sensible decisions to be made. These decisions can only be made through effective communications between managers, practitioners and those concerned with initial student education and continuing professional development. As clinical supervision becomes more acceptable in practice, we need to think creatively and draw on our experiences of roles that provide a critical safe space and offer support and guidance in the form of coaching and the use of positive feedback. But it is the practitioners who must play a major role in taking an appropriate course of action.

This will require sensitive handling and constructive debate about the type of support role as an appropriate mechanism for preparing professional practitioners in the early stages of their education programmes and as they continue in their careers. It is our view that we should begin to look closely at the support we provide for all staff with a view to involving clinical practitioners, managers, researchers and educators in the deliberations. Only then will we have a supportive, enabling culture that recognises and values clinical supervision, as well as acknowledging:

> 'Learning to reason productively can be emotional – even painful. But the pay off is great.'

> (Argyris, 1991, p. 107)

In moving clinical supervision from the presumptions to the practicalities, it may be useful now to consider and apply our experiences in addressing the questions that are commonly raised by practitioners in workshops, in everyday conversations and in practice.

Clinical supervision in practice: some common questions

(1) What is different about clinical supervision – 'we are doing it already'

As can be seen by the previous discussion in this chapter, clinical supervision essentially focuses on clinical practice and provides support and development within a relationship of mutual trust. It is an enabling partnership where you can constructively think about your practice, the care you give and the issues that cause you concern, as well as celebrating when things are going well. It is also important within such a relationship that you share good practice and begin to explore the assumptions that you make about your practice and how you work with others, as this will help you to value what you do.

You probably feel overloaded with the formal, informal and *ad hoc* meetings that impact on your work, and do not wish to consider adding to what may already be a busy working day. However, if you analyse these meetings you may find that they often revolve around the needs of others – the patients/clients, relatives and your colleagues. Clinical supervision provides a personal, safe space for you to think about your personal and professional needs and can play a significant part in helping you learn from experience by providing effective professional support. You will benefit from this type of relationship if you work in increasingly complex situations, where others' expectations are high, and the previously acknowledged informal support systems of collegial meetings or networking in the meal breaks, have diminished or been lost completely (Northcott, 1998b).

It may be that you are indeed having clinical supervision because your Trust or health centre has implemented such a system. In some cases that we know of, nothing formal has been introduced but nurses, midwives and health visitors have decided that they require regular meetings where they can focus on practice and professional performance within a group, or on an individual basis to critically analyse their work. However, from our discussions with practitioners, many do still think that they are having some form of clinical supervision even if they are engaging in general conversations with colleagues or superficially recalling certain situations or incidents with their peers.

We believe clinical supervision is about valuing yourself in the workplace and coping with the increasing demands that are placed upon you, allowing time out to think about and analyse what you are doing in attempting to deliver a good standard of care. The questions to ask yourself are:

- What do I believe clinical supervision is about?
- Can I make a case to support the view that I am doing it already'?

(2) What should we record and who keeps the records?

You should record what you want to record and you can do this in a structured way by keeping a reflective diary or professional development journal which can be included in your portfolio, if you have started to keep one as part of the PREP requirements. The key questions concerning record keeping are:

- Why do you want to keep a record?
- What do you want to record?
- What benefits will you get from keeping a record of your sessions?

You may be asked to make a commitment by signing a learning contract or written agreement with your supervisor to demonstrate that you are both committed to the process. In some organisations you may be asked to sign a record of each session but this only provides information that a session has taken place.

The responsibility for maintaining records is yours but it is a very useful exercise and an important part of learning from experience if you make regular notes after each session and reflect on them to make sense of what you shared, and what it says about you and your practice. Any records you decide to keep are of course confidential and they belong to you. However, we have found that if practitioners make time to jot down their feelings, or events that went well or badly, and analyse them, they benefit significantly. Such deliberations may inform the next session or may even be shared later with your clinical supervisor if you so wish.

Hopefully the days are gone when unnecessary records and documentation were produced to lie unused and unobtainable in locked filing cabinets. It is important in the record keeping process to use and work with your written reflections and see them as a viable aspect of your personal learning.

(3) What about confidentiality? .*

This is a common question that taxes practitioners at all levels but particularly those who are preparing to become supervisors for the first time. The reflective questions about confidentiality are:

- How would you like the information that you share to be handled?
- What would you do if someone shared something that was considered dangerous practice?

It is usual for the issues of confidentiality to be discussed and agreed between the clinical supervisor and practitioner when they set the ground rules or guidelines for how the relationship is to work. What is important, as you will appreciate when considering how you would wish to be treated, is that confidentiality should be strictly applied. Any disclosure of information should only normally occur if information is revealed within a session that indicates:

- A breach of the UKCC Code of Professional Practice
- A breach of law
- Serious exploitation or endangerment to others.

In such circumstances it is only right that the practitioner should be informed if the clinical supervisor makes the decision to disclose information to another source.

(4) What happens if I don't get on with my supervisor?

This is an often asked question but in our experience we have rarely had problems in this area, although of course personality clashes and the like do happen. As was explored in the mentoring case studies at the end of Chapter 3, sometimes circumstances and individuals do not gel.

The question to be asked here is:

- What do you think should happen?

There are several options open to individuals in situations where there are problems in the relationship, and as a general maxim we have found it useful not to encourage an early separation. We have observed that some of the best and most fruitful relationships have come about from meetings that initially have not appeared to go well. Often we have found that working out differences and coming to a shared understanding of what is valued and what is not, can engender some common areas of atgreement and mutual respect for each other's position which lead to eventual compatibility.

However, if there is no hope of obtaining a working partnership then other options have to come into play. Many of the Trust policies that we have scrutinised contain information on what to do in the event of a relationship that is not really working. If unresolved conflicts remain it is sensible to seek guidance from those identified to offer such support and advice, and in some cases this will be a nominated staff supervisor or clinical supervisor coordinator, in others it will be a designated manager. As a final resort – and we stress this – if all else, fails an individual can turn to the appropriate Trust policies on handling disputes and grievances.

(5) Who supports the supervisors?

It is an interesting question and relevant to ensuring an enabling health care culture where clinical supervision and the other professional learning support relationships can flourish. The questions that assist your deliberations are:

● How can the supervisors be supported?
● How can this support be effected in practice?

It is apparent from the emerging evidence concerning clinical supervision and how such relationships may work in practice, that the culture has to be an enabling one that encourages learning and proactivity in the workplace. Encouraging everyone involved to engage in some form of relationship that supports, develops and offers a safe space for thinking about and commenting on practice, would go some way towards promoting such a culture.

It may well be that clinical supervisors get together at regular intervals with their own supervisor within an individual, group or peer relationship style of supervision. Of course organisational demands, constraints and the distribution of resources, human, financial and mechanical, have to be taken into account, but it is important that supervisors are also supported and expected to critically examine their own practice. It is also essential that they are bound by the same realms of confidentiality that you are, and in this way trust can be built within the organisation.

(6) What skills do I require?

By now you know what question to expect to help you think about this:

● What skills do you think you require?

This is an important starting point because not all of us start at the same level of ability, understanding or skills and it is essential to explore and appreciate what you have, before you consider what you need to have to become a clinical supervisor or practitioner.

The wealth of interpersonal and enabling qualities are evident to us as we work with health care practitioners across the country that exist (see Chapter 2 for examples of these). Of course not everyone is an enabler or good communicator, but there is an issue here about whether those who are the 'disablers' should become clinical supervisors; certainly they may benefit from sampling effective clinical supervision themselves.

We have found that the most able clinical supervisors are those who:

- Command respect
- Are knowledgeable about practice
- Are eager to share ideas
- Are willing to learn from others.

It is also important that practitioners have responsibilities when engaging in clinical supervision and this requires individuals who:

- Are interested in practice development
- Are willing to assess their own performance
- Welcome the opportunity to share their thoughts and feelings about practice.

These are attributes and qualities that fit with Proctor's (1986) perspective that you will:

- Want to monitor your performance
- Wish to learn to develop competence
- Respond to support and encouragement.

The rest is up to you!

(7) Should I engage in individual or group supervision?

To make an informed choice it is essential to appreciate the different styles available, which are well documented in the literature, and having some understanding of these will allow you to reflect on:

- What clinical supervision do I want to engage in?
- What style will suit my individual needs?
- What other factors will influence my choice?

It is important in your search to find a style of supervision relationship that suits you personally, as well as fitting into your organisational structures and systems. Once again organisational demands, constraints, barriers and the availability of resources have to be taken into consideration. The main point is to match your personal needs with the organisational resources available, if you are to be successful in your selection.

Houston (1990) offers helpful considerations of supervision relationships, including:

- One to one sessions with a clinical supervisor from your own professional tribe (intraprofessional)
- One to one sessions with a clinical supervisor from another professional tribe (interprofessional)
- One to one peer supervision between practitioners of similar status and expertise
- Group supervision with sessions for individuals working together from the same profession (intraprofessional)
- Group supervision with sessions for individuals working together from different professions (interprofessional).

It has always fascinated us that some individuals who identify that they find difficulties relating one to one, should imagine that clinical supervision will be easier within a group. Certainly group supervision appears to work well in community and health visiting practice (drawing the intraprofessional tribes together) and in certain mental health and learning disability settings. In other examples that we know of, groups of clinical nurse specialists have organised their own group supervision sessions and employed someone from outside the group (and in some cases from a different tribe or discipline) to facilitate their sessions.

It is important here to consider that while working in a group can be exciting and fulfilling, it is beneficial to have some knowledge of group dynamics and how groups work, to get the best from this style of supervision. As you will know from your answers to the questions posed at the start of this section, the choice is entirely up to you, your particular needs and your relevant expertise, and is dependent on the resources that are available to you at the time of making your commitment.

(8) How will I know if clinical supervision is working?

This is not left until last because it is less important. Indeed assessing whether you are engaged in a worthwhile activity is a vital part of professional practice, but we have ended with this question because it is the one that raises many other interesting questions that should make you think more deeply about clinical supervision.

As part of an evaluative approach, which should illuminate the processes you are engaged in, we offer a set of evaluative questions, organised into different phases to offer structure to your deliberations and to encourage you to access them at different stages depending on your individual needs.

Phase 1: Preparing for clinical supervision

- Why am I engaging in clinical supervision?
- What do I want from the relationship?
- What areas of my practice do I want to develop?
- How can I successfully become involved?
- How will I know what I have gained or learnt from the experience?

Phase 2: Choosing a clinical supervisor

- What do I want from a clinical supervisor?
- Who has the skills to help me assess my limitations and build on my strengths?
- Who can help me challenge my assumptions?
- Who can I work effectively with?

Phase 3: Working with my clinical supervisor

- What are our mutual expectations of roles?
- What will be our commitment?
- How are we building trust and confidence in each other's abilities?
- Who sets the agenda?
- How does the relationship offer scope for my personal and professional development?

Phase 3: Reflecting on the relationship

- How do I feel about working with my clinical supervisor?
- How do I demonstrate that I remain committed to the clinical supervision process?
- What are the benefits and outcomes for patient/client care?
- Is ours an effective relationship and what criteria for effectiveness do we use?
- How will we know when these criteria have been met?
- How am I documenting what is happening and what am I learning?

It is suggested that these reflective activities will help you identify, and then work with further, the issues that arise – issues and challenges that will be particular to your own specific context and personal circumstances. It is is important that the dialogue that you begin to have with these questions is recorded in your portfolio, and may even be shared with your clinical supervisor if you should so wish.

Of course there are many other interesting and challenging questions that you can ask, but if you don't start somewhere, and continue with a 'spirit of inquiry', you will have trouble making sense of your increasingly complicated world.

References

Argyris, C. (1991) Teaching smart people to learn. *Harvard Business Review*, May–June, 99-109.

Atherton, T. (1999) *How to be Better at Delegation and Coaching*. Routledge, London.

Atkins, S. & Murphy, K. (1993) Reflection: a review of the literature. *Journal of Advanced Nursing*, **18**, 1188–92.

Audit Commission (1999) *First Assessment: A review of District Nursing Services in England & Wales*. Audit Commission Publications, Oxford.

Barnett, R. (1992) *Learning to Effect*. Society for Research into Higher Education, Open University Press, Buckingham.

Benner, P. (1984) *From Novice to Expert: Excellence and power in clinical nursing practice*. Addison Wesley, California.

Bines, H. & Watson, D. (1992) *Developing Professional Education*. Society for Research into Higher Education and Open University Press, Buckingham.

Bishop, V. (1994) Clinical supervision for an accountable profession. *Nursing Times*, **90** (39), 35–7.

Bishop, V. (ed.) (1998) *Clinical Supervision in Practice. Some questions, answers and guidelines*. Macmillan Press Ltd, Basingstoke.

Bond, M. & Holland, S. (1998) *Clinical Supervision for Nurses*. Open University Press, Buckingham.

Boud, D. & Walker, N. (1996) Barriers to Reflection on Experience. In: *Using Experience for Learning*, (eds D. Boud, R. Cohen & D. Walker). Society for Research into Higher Education and Open University Press, Buckingham.

Boud, D., Keogh, R. & Walker, D. (1985) *Reflection: Turning Experience into Learning*. Kogan Page, London.

Brady, T. (1998) Spare us the pretentious practice of reflecting. *Nursing Times*, letters, **94** (9), 24.

Brookfield, S.D. (1987) *Developing Critical Thinkers. Challenging adults to explore alternative ways of thinking and acting*. Open University Press, Milton Keynes.

Brown, R. (1995) *Portfolio Development and Profiling for Nurses*, 2nd edn. Quay Books, Salisbury, Wilts.

Burnard, P. (1988) Mentors: a supporting act. *Nursing Times*, **84** (66), 27–8.

Burnard, P (1989) Developing critical ability in nurse education. *Nurse Education Today*, **9**, 271–5.

Butterworth, T. (1998) Clinical supervision as an emerging idea in nursing. In: *Clinical Supervision and Mentorship in Nursing*, (eds T. Butterworth, J. Faugier & P. Burnard). Stanley Thornes (Publishers) Ltd, London.

Butterworth, T. & Faugier, J. (1992) *Clinical Supervision and Mentorship in Nursing*. Chapman Hall, London.

Butterworth, T., Bishop, V. & Carson, J. (1996) First steps towards evaluating clinical supervision in nursing and health visiting. 1. Theory, policy and practice development. A review. *Journal of Clinical Nursing*, **5**, 127–32.

Butterworth, T., Faugier, J. & Burnard, P. (eds) (1998) *Clinical Supervision and Mentorship in Nursing*. Stanley Thornes (Publishers) Ltd, London.

Cahill, H.A. (1996) A qualitative analysis of student nurses' perceptions of mentorship. *Journal of Advanced Nursing*, **24**, 791–9.

Cameron, E. (1998) *Facilitation Made Easy. Practical Tips to Improve facilitation in workshops*. Routledge, London.

Carr, E.C.J. (1996) Reflecting on clinical practice: hectoring talk or reality? *Journal of Clinical Nursing*, **5**, 289–95.

Carter, E.M.A. (1993) Measuring the Returns. In: *The Return of the Mentor. Strategies for workplace learning*, (eds B.B. Caldwell & E.M.A. Carter). The Falmer Press, London.

Chief Nursing Officer (1994) *Clinical supervision*, CNO Professional Letter **94** (5). DoH, London.

Clarke, R. & Croft, P. (1998) *Critical Reading for the Reflective Practitioner. A Guide for Primary Care*. Butterworth-Heinemann, Oxford.

Clothier, C., MacDonald, C.A. & Shaw, D.A. (1994) *Independent Inquiry into Death and Injuries on the Children's Ward at Grantham Kresteven General Hospital During the Period February to April 1991* (The Allitt Inquiry). HMSO, London.

Cox, R. (1992) Learning Theory and Professional Life. *Media and Technology for Human Development*, **4** (4), 217–32.

Crouch, S. (1991) Critical Incident Analysis. *Nursing*, (37), 30–31.

Cutcliffe, J.R. & Proctor, B. (1998) An alternative training approach to clinical supervision: 1. *British Journal of Nursing*, **7** (5), 280–85.

Dale, M. (1998) *Developing Management Skills*. Routledge, London.

Dartington, A. (1994) Where angels fear to tread. Idealism, despondency and inhibition of thought in hospital nursing. In: *The Unconscious at Work*, (eds A. Obholzer & V.Z. Roberts). Routledge, London.

Davies, C. (1976) Experience of dependency and control in work; the case of nurses. *Journal of Advanced Nursing*, **1**, 273–82.

Davies, C. (1995) *Gender and the Professional Predicament in Nursing*. Buckingham, Open University Press.

Davies, N. (1993) *Murder on Ward Four*. Chatto & Windus, London.

Davies, P. (1993) Value Yourself. *Nursing Times*, **89** (4), 52.

Dewey, J. (1938) *Experience and Education*. Collier, New York.

DoH (1993) *A Vision for the Future. The Nursing Midwifery and Health Visiting Contribution to Health & Health Care*. Department of Health, London.

DoH (1998) *A First Class Service: quality in the NHS*. Department of Health, London.

DoH (1999) *Clinical Governance. Quality in the NHS*. NHS Management Executive, Department of Health, Leeds.

Dolan, T. (1998) Collaboration and partnership. *Nursing Times – Learning Curve*, **2** (1), 4–5.

Driscoll, J. (2000) *Practising Clinical Supervision – A Reflective Approach.* Balliere Tindall/RCN, London.

Earwaker, J. (1992) *Helping and Supporting Students. Rethinking the Issues.* The Society for Research into Higher Education and Open University Press, Buckingham.

ENB (1994) *Using your portfolio: A Resource for Practitioners.* ENB Publications, London.

ENB (1988) *Institutional and Course Approval/Reapproval Process, Information Required – Criteria and Guidelines.* 1988/39/APS. ENB, London.

Eraut, M. (1994) *Developing Professional Knowledge and Competence.* Faber Press, London.

Farrington, A. (1995) Models of clinical supervision. *British Journal of Nursing,* **4** (15), 87–9.

Faugier, J. (1998) The supervisory relationship. In: *Clinical Supervision and Mentorship in Nursing,* (eds T. Butterworth, J. Faugier & Burnard). Stanley Thornes (Publishers) Ltd, London.

Fournies, F.F (1978) *Coaching for improved work performance.* Van Nostrand Reinhold, New York.

Freire, P. (1972) *Pedagogy of the Oppressed.* Penguin, Harmondsworth.

Fish, D. & Twinn, S. (1997) *Quality Clinical Supervision in the Health Care Professions. Principled Approaches to Practice.* Butterworth-Heinemann, London.

Fisher, M. (1996) Using reflective practice in clinical supervision. *Professional Nurse,* **11** (7), 443–4.

Fowler, J. & Chevannes, M. (1998) Evaluating the efficacy of reflective practice within the context of clinical supervision. *Journal of Advanced Nursing,* **27,** 379–82.

GLPQ, (1997) *Guidance for Candidates on Preparation and Submission of Portfolios.* Greater London Post Qualifying Education and Training Consortium, London.

Graham, I.W. (1995) Reflective practice; using the action learning group mechanism. *Nurse Education Today,* **15,** 28–32.

Gulland, A. (1999) What is Clinical Governance? *Nursing Times,* **95** (9), 17.

Hawkins, P. & Shohet, R. (1989) *Supervision in the Helping Professions.* Open University Press, Milton Keynes.

Heron, J. (1977) *Dimensions of Facilitation Style.* Human Research Project. Department of Adult Education, University of Surrey, Guildford.

Heron, J. (1999) *The Complete Facilitators Handbook.* Routledge, London.

Hill, J. (1989) Supervision in the caring professions: a literature review. *Community Psychiatric Nursing Journal,* **9** (5), 9–15.

Horton, M. (1990) *The Long Haul.* Doubleday, New York.

Houston, G. (1990) *Supervision and Counselling.* The Rochester Foundation, London.

Hudson-Jones, A. (ed.) (1988) *Images of Nurses: Perspectives from History, Art, Literature.* University of Pennsylvania Press, Philadelphia.

Hughes L. & Pengelly, P. (1997) *Staff Supervision in a Turbulent Environment.* Jessica Kingsley Publishers, London.

Hull, C. & Redfern, L. (1996) *Profiles and Portfolios for Nurses and Midwives.* Macmillan, London.

Inskipp, F. & Proctor, B. (1993) *The Art, Craft and Tasks of Supervision. Part 1: Making the Most of Supervision.* Cascade publications, Twickenham.

James, C.R. (1990) *Developing portfolio-based learning.* Paper presentation to the Steering Committee, *Nursing Times.* Open Learning, Macmillan, London,

James, C.R. & Clarke, B.A. (1994) Reflective practice in nursing: issues and implications for nurse education. *Nurse Education Today,* **14,** 82–90.

Jasper, M.A. (1998) Using portfolios to advance practice. In: *Advanced Nursing Practice,* (eds G. Rolfe & P. Fullbrook). Butterworth-Heinemann, Oxford.

J.M. Consulting (1998) The regulation of nurses, midwives and health visitors. *Report on a review of the Nurses, Midwives and Health Visitors Act 1997.* J.M. Consulting, Bristol.

Johns, C. (1993) Professional supervision. *Journal of Nursing Management,* **1,** 9–18.

Johns, C. & Graham, J. (1996) Using a reflective model of nursing and guided reflection. *Nursing Standard,* **11,** 2, 34–8.

Jones, A. (1995) Taking Counsel. *Nursing Times,* **91** (26), 28–9.

Jowett. S., Walton, I. & Payne, S. (1994) *Challenges and Change in Nurse Education – A study of the implementation of Project 2000.* National Federation for Educational Research, Berkshire.

Kadushin, A. (1976) *Supervision in Social Work.* Columbia University Press, New York.

Kelly, K.J. (1992) *Nursing Staff Development. Current Competence Future Focus.* J. B. Lippincott, Philadelphia.

Knight, J.F. & Scott, W. (1998) *A Practical Guide to Using Partnerships in Facilitation.* Routledge, London.

Knowles, M.S. (1984) *Andragogy in Action: Applying Modern Principles of Adult Learning.* Jossey-Bass, San Francisco.

Kohner, N. (ed) (1994) *Clinical Supervision in Practice.* Kings Fund Centre. Bournemouth English Book Centre, Dorset.

Kolb, D. A. (1984) *Experiential Learning.* Prentice Hall, New Jersey.

L'Aiguaille, Y. (1994) In: *Reflective Practice in Nursing: The Growth of the Reflective Practitoner,* (eds A.M. Palmer, S. Burns & C. Bulman). Blackwell Science, Oxford.

Maben, J. & Macleod Clark, J. (1997) The impact of Project 2000. *Nursing Times,* **93** (35), 55–8.

Maggs, C. (1998) Introducing clinical supervision and beginning evaluation. In: *Clinical Supervision in Practice. Some Questions, Answers and Guidelines,* (ed. V. Bishop). Macmillan Press Ltd, Basingstoke.

Marchant, H. (1986) Supervision a training perspective. In: *Enabling and Ensuring,* (eds M. Marken & M. Payne.) Council for Education and Training in Youth and Community Work, London.

Marrow, C.E., MaCauley, D.M. & Crumbie, A. (1997) Promoting reflective practice through structured clinical supervision. *Journal of Nursing Management,* **5,** 77–82.

McCallion, H. & Baxter, T. (1995) Clinical supervision – how it works in the real world. *Nursing Management*, **1**, (9) 20–21.

McCoppin, Gardner, H. (1994) *Tradition and Reality*. Churchill Livingstone, Melbourne.

McCormack, B. & Hopkins, E. (1995) The development of clinical leadership through supported reflective practice. *Journal of Clinical Nursing*, 4, 161–8.

McEvoy, P. (1993) A Chance for Feedback. *Nursing Times*, **89** (47), 52–5.

McGrowther, J. (1995) *Profiles, Portfolios and How to Build Them*. Scutari Press, London.

Miller, N. & Boud, D. (1996) Animating Learning from Experience. In: *Working with Experience. Animating Learning*, (eds D. Boud & N. Miller). Routledge, London.

Mitchell, P. & Shaw, T. (1994) A guide to profiling and portfolios. *Nursing Standard*, **8** (41), 25–8.

Mockford, C.D. (1994) The use of peer group review in the assessment of project work in higher education. *Mentoring and Tutoring*, **2** (2), 45–52.

Moore, C. & Carter, J. (1998) Exploration of the empowering potential of clinical supervision, reflected and action research. In: *Transforming Nursing Through Reflective Practice*, (eds C. Johns & D. Freshwater). Blackwell Science, Oxford.

Morton-Cooper, A. (1998) *Preceptorship via action research; a reflective account*. Doctoral thesis, Continuing Education Centre, the University of Warwick.

Morton-Cooper, A. & Bamford, M. (1997) *Excellence in Health Care Management*. Blackwell Science, Oxford.

Muir Gray, J.M. (1997) *Evidence-based Health Care. How to Make Health Policy and Management Decisions*. Churchill Livingstone, London.

NHS Executive (1998) *Consultation on a Strategy for Nursing, Midwifery and Health Visiting*. Health Service Circular 1998/045. NHS Executive, London.

Nicklin, P (1995) Super supervision. *Nursing Management*, **2** (5), 24–5.

Nicklin, P (1997) A practice-centred model of clinical supervision. *Nursing Times*, **93** (46), 52–4.

Norman, S. (1998) Postscript: Supporting the initiative: the role of the UKCC. In: *Clinical Supervision in Practice. Some Questions, Answers and Guidelines*, (ed. V. Bishop). Macmillan Press Ltd, Basingstoke.

Northcott, N. (1998a) The development of guidelines on clinical supervision in clinical practice settings. In: *Clinical Supervision in Practice. Some Questions, Answers and Guidelines*, (ed. V. Bishop). Macmillan Press Ltd, Basingstoke.

Northcott, N. (1998b) Don't accept the debrief. *Nursing Times*, **94** (10), 32.

Ogier, M.E. (1989) *Working and Learning: The Learning Environment in Clinical Learning*. Scutari Press, London.

Ogier, M.E. & Cameron-Buccheri, R. (1990) Supervision: a cross-cultural approach. *Nursing Standard*, **4** (31), 24–7.

Open University (1998) *Clinical Supervision: A Development Pack for Nurses*. School of Health & Social Welfare, The Open University, Milton Keynes.

Orton, H.D. (1981) Ward learning climates and student nurse responses. *Nursing Times*, Occasional paper, **77** (23), 65–8.

Palmer, E.A. (1987) *The nature of the mentor relationship in nurse education. A study to introduce the mentor.* Unpublished thesis, South Bank Polytechnic, London.

Palmer, A. (1992) *Open Learning: Issues for Educators.* Education Workshop – Quality in Education Conference, Manchester, The second *Nursing Times* Open Learning Conference.

Palmer, A. (1993) The *Nursing Times* Open Learning Programme: an innovation in collaboration and design. *The Annals of Community-Orientated Education*, **6**, 259–72.

Palmer, A. (1997) Learning to reflect. *Nursing Times Learning Curve*, **1** (2), 2–3.

Palmer, A. & Wilson, A. (1997) *Clinical supervision – pilot.* Report to the Task Group, Harefield Hospital NHS Trust.

Palmer, A.M., Burns, S. & Bulman, C. (1994) *Reflective Practice in Nursing: The Growth of the Reflective Practitioner.* Blackwell Science, Oxford.

Parsloe, E. (1995) Coaching, mentoring and assessing. *A Practical Guide to Developing Competencies*, revised edition. Kogan Page, London.

Payne, D. (1999) Vital links in the chain. *Nursing Times*, **95** (10), 15.

Pietroni, R. & Millard, L. (1996) Portfilio based learning. In: Professional Development in General Practice, (eds J. Hasler & D. Pendleton). Open University Press, Buckingham.

Pietroni, R. & Palmer, A. (1994) *Handy hints for portfolio-based learning.* Course document, the MA Continuing Professional Education (Health and Social Care). The Centre for Community Care & Primary Health, University of Westminster, London.

Pietroni, R. & Palmer, A. (1995) Portfolio based learning and the role of mentors. *Education for General Practice*, **6**, 111–14.

Platt-Koch, L.M. (1986) Clinical supervision for psychiatric nurses. *Journal of Psycho-Social Nursing*, **26** (1), 7–15.

Pritchard, J. (ed) (1995) *Good Practice in Supervision. Statutory and Voluntary Organisations.* Jessica Kingsley Publishers, London.

Proctor, B. (1986) A cooperative exercise in accountability. In: *Enabling and Ensuring*, (eds M. Marken & M. Payne). Council for Education and Training in Youth and Community Work, London.

Ramsden, P. (1992) *Learning to Teach in Higher Education.* Routledge, London.

Rich, A. & Parker, D. (1995) Reflection & critical incident analysis: ethical & moral implications of their use within and midwifery education. *Journal of Advanced Nursing*, 22, 1050–57.

Rickards, T. (1992) *How to Win as a Mature Student.* Kogan Page, London.

Rogers, C.R. (1969) *Freedom to Learn.* Charles E. Merrill Publishing Co, Columbus, Ohio.

Rolfe, G. (1998) Beyond expertise: reflective and reflexive nursing practice. In: *Transforming Nursing Through Reflective Practice*, (eds C. Johns & D. Freshwater). Blackwell Science, Oxford.

Routledge, J., Wilson, M., MacArthur, M., Richardson, B. & Stephenson, R. (1997)

Reflection on the development of a reflective assessment. *Medical Teacher*, **19** (2), 122–8.

Sadler, P. (1989) Management development. In: *Personnel Management in Britain*, (ed. K. Sissons). Blackwell Science, Oxford.

Salvage, J. (1998) Clinical Supervision – comment. *Nursing Times*, **94** (23), 24.

Schon, D.A. (1983) *The Reflective Practitioner: How Professionals Think in Action*. Basic Books, New York.

Schon, D.A. (1988) *Educating the Reflective Practitioner. Toward a new design for Teaching and Learning in the Professions*. Jossey-Bass, London.

Simosko, S. (1991) *APL: A Practical Guide for Professionals*. Kogan Page, London.

Spouse, J. (1996) The effective mentor: a model for student-centred learning. *Nursing Times*, **92** (13), 32–5.

Swierings, J. & Wierdsma, A. (1992) *Becoming a Learning Organisation – Beyond the Learning Curve*. Addison Wesley Publishers, Wokingham.

Taylor, R.B. (1980) The role of the Academic Adviser. *Journal of Medical Education*, **55**, 216–17.

Teasdale, K. (1996) Using personal profiles in reflective practice. *Professional Nurse*, **11** (5), 323–4.

Tichen, A. & Binnie, A. (1995) The art of clinical supervision. *Journal of Clinical Nursing*, **4**, 327–34.

Tomlinson, P. (1995) Understanding Mentoring: Reflective Strategies for School-based Teacher Education. Open University Press, Buckingham.

Topping, K.J. (1994) Organising peer tutoring in higher and further education. Part 1: introduction, targeting, selection, logistics and resources. *Mentoring and Tutoring*, **2** (2), 11–18.

Tsang, N.M. (1998) Re-examining reflection – a common issue of professional concern in social work, teacher and nursing education. *Journal of Inter-professional Care*, **12** (1), 21–31.

UKCC (1986) *Project 2000: A New Preparation for Practice*. UKCC, London.

UKCC (1995) *Fact Sheet 4: Your Personal Professional Profile*. UKCC, London.

UKCC (1996) *Position Statement on Clinical Supervision for Nursing & Health Visiting*. UKCC, London.

University of London (1992) *Roles and responsibilities of Academic Advisers*. Student Handbook, MA Higher & Professional Education. Centre for Higher Education Studies, London.

van den Brink-Budgen, R. (1996) *Critical Thinking for Students*. How to Books Ltd, Plymouth.

Wallace, D. (1996) Experiential learning and critical thinking in nursing. *Nursing Standard*, **10** (31), 43–7.

Weil, S. (1998) Rhetorics and realities in public service organisations: systematic practice and organisational learning as critically reflexive action research (CRAR). *Systematic Practice and Action Research*, **11** (1), 37–61.

Weil, S. & McGill, I. (eds) (1989) *Making Sense of Experiential Learning: Diversity and Theory and Practice*. Society for Research into Higher Education & Open University, Buckingham.

Weightman, J. (1996) *Managing People in the Health Service*. Institute of Personnel and Development. Cromwell Press, Wiltshire.

Westheimer, I.J. (1977) *The Practice of Supervision in Social Work. A Guide for Staff Supervisors*. Ward Lock Educational, London.

White, E. (1996) Clinical supervision and Project 2000: The identification of some substantive issues. *Nursing Times Research*, **1** (2), 102–11.

Wilkin, P., Bowers, L. & Monk, J. (1997) Clinical supervision: managing the resistance. *Nursing Times*, **93** (8), 48–9.

Williams, P.A. (1998) Using theories of professional knowledge and reflective practice to influence educational change. *Medical Teacher*, **20** (1), 28–34.

Wilson, A. & Palmer, A. (1998) *The Outcomes and Benefits of Clinical Supervision – Interim Evaluation Report*. Harrow & Hillingdon Healthcare NHS Trust, Middlesex.

Wilson, A. & Palmer, A. (1999) *Making Clinical Supervision Work: The Evaluation Report*. Harrow & Hillingdon Healthcare NHS Trust, Middlesex.

Wilson-Barnett, J., Butterworth, T., White, E., Twinn, S., Davies, S. & Riley, L. (1995) Clinical support and the Project 2000 nursing student: factors influencing this process. *Journal of Advanced Nursing*, **21**, 1152–8.

Wolsey, P. & Leach, L. (1997) Clinical supervision: a hornet's nest? *Nursing Times*, **93** (44), 24–7.

Wright, S., Elliot, M. & Scholfield, H. (1997) A networking approach to clinical supervision. *Nursing Standard*, **11** (18), 30–41.

Yates, P., Cunningham, J., Moyle, W. & Wolin, J. (1997) Peer mentorship in clinical education: outcomes of a pilot programme for first year students. *Nurse Education Today*, 17, 508–14.

Chapter 5
Providing a Professional Support Framework

'The art of medicine, of being a good doctor, or being
a good nurse – I guess it's probably the art of being
good at anything – is judgment, of actually knowing
where your skills, where your knowledge ends, and
knowing when to seek help elsewhere.'

(Medical Director of an NHS Trust (SCOPME, 1999)

Introduction

The concepts of mentoring, preceptorship and clinical supervision have
been fully explored in the earlier chapters and our intentions here are to
make a case for effective support provision and tease out the differences
between the three significant support roles that have been identified as
being the mainstay of any professional support framework. Although
intended primarily for nurses, midwives and health visitors, it could be
easily adapted to provide a framework of support for others involved in
health care, where similar professional entrances and routes exist.

The confusion in roles

In many areas and in British nursing and midwifery in particular, mentoring has been used extensively and often inappropriately for student
support and assessment, as explored in Chapters 2 and 4. Difficulties
arose which will have become apparent as you have read through this
book and as the complexities of mentoring, preceptorship and clinical
supervision have been unravelled.

Student nurses and student midwives now have access to personal
tutors, are assessed by assessors and facilitated by mentors, and in some
instances all these complex roles with their individual responsibilities
and possible conflicts are expected to be carried out by one qualified

practitioner. In many cases the preparation is adequate but in others it remains, at best, rudimentary, without exploration of the underpinning theoretical deliberations that continue to surface and are being debated.

It can come as no surprise that there is lack of understanding and confusion with attempts made to bypass the real issues by inventing other labels. We have noted the continued rise in the different terms used for identifying those who support students through their educational programmes and practice placements. Besides the more readily recognisable labels already documented in this chapter, 'key worker', 'facilitator–aide', 'clinical supporter', 'supervisor–mentor' are the more interesting and colourful titles found.

We could add one more to the growing list: 'prementorvisor', an honorary title for those who are attempting to come to terms with being appointed to provide clinical support. They are called mentors, function as preceptors and think they might quite like to be clinical supervisors. They have to teach, support, coach, assess and supervise students as they themselves, often in new posts, have to cope with the demands of their practice, taking responsibility for their own continuing professional development and by the nature of their caring profession, meeting the needs of patients, clients, customers or consumers. No wonder there is confusion, with practitioners distrustful of any new suggestions. Table 5.1 offers an overview of the more readily recognisable professional roles in practice.

Role comparisons

What may have confused those planning the implementation of professional learning support roles in the past, is that mentoring, preceptorship and clinical supervision relationships appear to possess many of the same inherent qualities and characteristics. This would be expected as all three provide enabling, supportive relationships and, as can be seen from the previous chapters, there are similarities in approach which, in the past, have caused managers and educators difficulties in making a clear distinction between the roles, causing them to be used indiscriminately and inappropriately.

In examining the enabling components it becomes evident that there are core characteristics common to the different support roles and these are identified as:

- Motivating individuals to set their own agenda for learning and practising
- Providing safe opportunities for critical reflection
- Advising, counselling and guiding

Table 5.1 Glossary of learning support roles in the professional domain. This is not intended to be exhaustive and as the debate about support roles develops and new understandings emerge, so will our interpretations of what is available.

Assessor	A professionally competent practitioner who is prepared in the skills required to assess the performance of another.
Clinical supervisor	A professional practitioner who provides an interactive professional partnership, where there is shared responsibility for stimulating critical reflection, reviewing and assessing personal performance, as well as providing support and emotional refreshment.
Coach	A skilled practitioner who provides an understanding of the nature of professional practice, through the provision of learning opportunities and supportive intervention. Coaching involves constructive monitoring and feedback of performance to aid learning and personal development, allowing the student to practise effectively.
Co-tutoring	Individual practitioners are encouraged to work together in pairs or small groups to assist each other's learning and to provide constructive feedback and personal support.
Mentor	Someone who provides an enabling relationship that facilitates another's personal growth and development. The relationship is dynamic, reciprocal and can be emotionally intense. Within such a relationship the mentor assists with career development and guides the mentee through the organisational, social and political networks.
Peer, peer pals, buddy	Someone considered a colleague of equal status, forming a collaborative relationship that is mutual and non competitive. A peer group as a collection of peers can provide an informal, supportive network acting as colleagues and friends.
Preceptor	An identified experienced practitioner who provides transitional role support within a collegial relationship.
Role model	This individual provides demonstrable behaviour that merits imitation and assists learning by example.

- Assisting individuals to learn through their successes and failures
- Being an effective role model
- Recognising and supporting an individual's strengths
- Developing capabilities by offering constructive feedback.

It is our suggestion that these enabling characteristics span the three significant professional support relationships and that other 'relationship-specific' enabling functions become apparent due to the particular nature of each relationship. This is demonstrated in the enabling functions of the mentor in Chapter 2, where the core enabling aspects are identified, with the inclusion of the more specific ones that relate particularly to mentoring. The specific enabling elements in this case are those of career socialisation, resource provision, the nature and degree of challenge and an awareness of leadership capabilities.

A further example was demonstrated within the checklist of key functions of the supervisor–coach in Chapter 4. In this manner clinical supervision can be considered to relate to the common enabling characteristics but the specific enabling aspects concern the development of clinical practice, quality assurance aspects and personal performance review.

Mentoring, preceptorship and clinical supervision provide an enabling relationship of some intensity, but the mentor relationship is one of closer, emotional intimacy. In making a comparison between mentoring and preceptorship, both Shapiro *et al.* (1978) and Puetz (1985) identified a continuum of roles that ranged from role modelling through preceptorship to mentoring. Figure 5.1 shows how the separate entities relate to each other in terms of the degree of intimacy required within the identified relationships. Until these early conceptualisations of the different roles, it was relatively easy to confuse functions and to experience difficulty in appreciating where the application of role modelling might fit with the more enabling roles of mentoring and preceptorship.

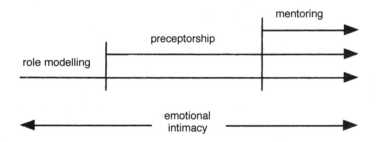

Fig. 5.1   Relationships of support roles.

Lack of clarity has also arisen because of a basic misrepresentation of the nature of the classical mentor and how, without due care and attention, it can be stripped of its essential qualities and reduced to a more simplified, functional relationship as that of contract mentoring. In this more formal type of mentoring relationship there emerge tasks and functions that resemble both preceptorship and clinical supervision, and the boundaries of the relationships overlap.

It remains important to recognise that the roles of mentoring, preceptorship and clinical supervision are complementary and of equal value in providing learning support and professional socialisation. This is further borne out by the work of Bond & Holland (1998) who recognise that the roles may vary in nature, duration, context and practical application but recommend that they all have a valuable part to play in assisting personal and professional development of individuals. Our intention here is to clarify the differences between mentoring and preceptorship, a process we commenced in the first edition, and then to consider where clinical supervision best fits.

The differences between mentoring and preceptorship

Clarification of the nature of the differences is offered by Deane & Campbell (1985) who in making a comparison of mentor and preceptor functions suggest that mentors take a specific, personal interest in assisting an individual practitioner with their career development. This enables the mentor to enhance career planning and encourage personal and professional satisfaction in those they are mentoring. To achieve this the mentor and mentee have to maintain close contact, meeting as need dictates, but they do not necessarily have to be working in close proximity or within the same clinical setting.

In comparison, preceptors 'act as agents for their employers, to assist other employees or students in adjusting to their new role' (Deane & Campbell, 1985, p. 144). It is also important that preceptors and preceptees work closely together to form a regular alliance at the time of role transition. This means working in partnership with structured objectives and clear expectations or outcomes for a specified duration, where there is an element of formal assessment in the form of 'objective processes for measuring achievement' (Deane & Campbell, 1985, p. 144). The resulting supportive, individualised teaching and learning interaction enables practitioners to develop their knowledge and skills within a trusting, supportive relationship.

Traditionally in the past the preceptor role in its application specifically for students, has come to represent that of the clinical practitioner who facilitates day-to-day practice, teaching and assessing while having clinical responsibilities. As identified in Chapter 3, this has been adapted by the UKCC and researchers within British nursing to relate to an experienced, registered practitioner who works in partnership with another newly registered, qualified practitioner (UKCC, 1995). The preceptor provides assistance and support in the process of learning and adaptation to new roles and situations in a variety of clinical environments, enabling transitional role support (Morton-Cooper, 1998). This description of preceptor function appears to fit well with the notion of preceptorship as suggested by Deane and Campbell's earlier considerations.

Mentoring is more personally directed to assist in setting a wider exposure to the world of work, while the preceptor in contrast, assists with practice development and clinical competence. The mentor may also assist with practical concerns at certain points in the duration of the relationship, but essentially the mentor is more concerned with professional development in terms of broader career issues.

A preceptor assists in the socialisation process but, once again, the role as it currently presents will be more functionally specific and related more particularly to the practitioner's needs in the clinical environment. In preceptorship the emphasis is on working towards the mutually agreed and established goals and outcomes set by the preceptor and practitioner. The mentor, by comparison, assists in widening an individual's personal network and helps with the social and professional introductions into the larger arena of professional practice.

Classical mentoring is determined by the natural partnership to provide unstructured learning support; however in preceptorship the basis for the relationship is structured learning support. The nature of this learning support is determined by the requirements of the organisation and the profession, framed within specified or structured outcomes which, of course, can and should be negotiated and mutually agreed.

In terms of the specified outcomes, some programmes of formal mentoring with specific outcomes and an over-reliance on structure, will blur the boundaries between the two roles as can be seen in Fig. 5.2. This diagram is adapted from Fig. 2.5, to further demonstrate the overlapping boundaries of both mentoring and preceptorship as applied to clinical practice. The resulting continuum illustrates the range of approaches, from classical mentoring through semi-structured formats to more structured applications of contract mentoring. As previously discussed this is mentoring at its most formal, and contract mentoring will include preparation programmes for mentors and mentees and random allocation and artificial matching of individuals, with specified goals and outcomes. This shifts the perspective towards that of preceptorship programmes and there may be some overlap in the nature and function of the relationships that result.

Exploring the continuum in Fig. 5.2 aids in identifying the artificial boundaries that exist between mentoring and preceptorship. The diagram demonstrates where mentoring – in its formal application in health care, with the assignment of contract mentors – crosses the boundary of the more clinically orientated, preceptor role. In contemplating such inter-relationships it becomes easier to appreciate how confusion has arisen as formal mentoring approaches were introduced into practice, and preceptorship programmes were subsequently developed, without due care to their specific roles and functions.

It is important to remember that classical mentoring is naturally

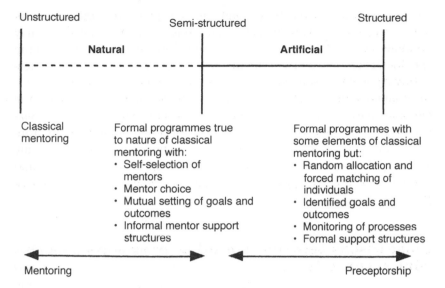

Fig. 5.2 The continuum of informality and formality, classical mentoring, formal mentoring and preceptorship.

determined by the individuals who enter into the relationship. Once mentoring programmes are constructed that have formally identified, set outcomes, monitoring elements, reliance on preparation as 'training for mentors', and approved support structures, the boundaries between mentoring and preceptorship become decidedly less distinct.

Evidence, both empirical and anecdotal, demonstrates and stresses the long term nature of classical mentoring relationships. The mentor has broader responsibilities for assisting in the personal and career development of those with whom they are in partnership. The complex and dynamic nature of the collaboration is dependent on the personal characteristics of each of the partners to sustain it through the peaks and troughs of a long term, essentially adaptive, relationship. As has been previously discussed in the section on mentoring, the duration of the relationship is set by the collaborating individuals.

For the mentoring process to be initiated and developed to its full potential, anything between two and fifteen years provides the expected lifespan for such relationships. This contrasts with the newly formulated ideas about preceptorship programmes in nursing, midwifery and health visiting, which are much more practice based and employer – or professionally – directed with a predetermined 'shelf life' of approximately four months.

In cases of classical mentoring, the practitioners select each other as previously stressed; however, in formal mentoring, selection or assigning of mentors may occur. In implementing preceptorship it appears likely that, due to work demands and shift patterns, individuals will continue to be identified and paired together for the duration of the specified programme of development.

Having begun to separate mentoring from preceptorship and identify the commonalities and the differences of the two support relationship, it becomes part of the current debate to consider where clinical supervision take its place within a framework of professional support. It is important to reiterate that all three relationships provide a safe space for support, development, reflection and learning in their own unique manner, and relative application of functions when applied in clinical practice.

Comparisons between mentoring, preceptorship and clinical supervision

Comparing clinical supervision and preceptorship appears relatively straightforward because the roles can be thought of as appropriately distinct and significantly different, in both application and function.

Preceptorship, as it is evolving in the UK, provides a transitional role support relationship with its well defined boundaries and focus on support for making the transition, be it returning to practice, changing role or responsibilities, or for the recently qualified, for taking the first tentative steps as a registered practitioner. This role is ideal for different professional and occupational groups and could so easily be transferred to provide professional support for junior doctors in training, GP registrars making the transition to general practice, or newly qualified physiotherapists and radiographers taking on their first departmental role on qualification. The role of the preceptor as explored in Chapter 3 has a significant part to play, recognising that it is a relatively short term relationship with well defined aims, outcomes and learning processes.

It may well be that in the future practitioners will be assigned a preceptor in the first instance on registration, and if the resulting relationship is successful, the same partnership can continue within a clinical alliance that assists with professional development and enables individual competence and critical reflection in practice. The resulting transition from preceptorship as an immediate resource to the longer term requirements of clinical supervision can then be readily acknowledged and recognised by those who will most benefit.

The main issue it appears to us, having made the distinction between mentoring and preceptorship previously, is in making a comparison between the more enabling relationships of mentoring and clinical supervision. Separating mentoring from clinical supervision is a some-what more difficult undertaking, particularly as mentoring has been variously described and distorted in practice, and clinical supervision is still emerging within a changing health service and adapting nursing culture.

To describe mentoring as solely career socialisation, clinical super-vision as clinical socialisation and preceptorship as transitional role support, would be an over simplification, even though this may initially help practitioners begin to reflect on how these professional support roles may fit together and each find their rightful place in practice. As described earlier in this chapter, within an adaptation of the construct first suggested by Puetz (1985), mentoring, preceptorship and role modelling can be linked and integrated by their overlapping functions, role definitions, responsibilities and levels of intimacy.

The potential relationship of clinical supervision, preceptorship and mentoring is illustrated in Fig. 5.3, to demonstrate the degree of inte-gration and intimacy which is a further adaptation of the previous deliberations. This illustration demonstrates where coaching and clin-ical supervision may well fit, as coaching is evident in mentoring rela-tionships as a facet of professional support and is substituted for the more passive element of role modelling. As discussed in the previous chapter, we make the case for considering coaching in relation to the clinical supervision relationship for students, when considering their specific practice needs.

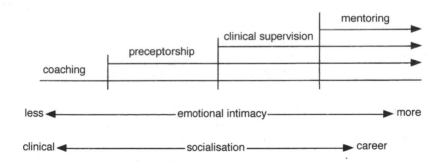

Fig. 5.3   Relationships of significant professional support roles.

It is difficult to make a clear distinction between clinical supervision and mentoring, and available research studies are difficult to interpret. There is evidence that the different definitions of the roles influence the respondents' views of what is occurring. Sands *et al.* (1991) report that in studies where the mentor is defined in broad terms as sponsor and helper, mentoring becomes more evident. However, comparative analysis of results remains a contentious issue and a difficult venture when findings are influenced by terminology and definition and where professional support roles are used interchangeably (Wilson-Barnett *et al.*, 1995; White, 1996).

If mentoring is defined and associated with the apprenticeship mode of operating, as can be seen in some of the initial teacher training initiatives, then the resulting relationship becomes significantly more aligned with the more instructional forms of support like coaching (Adams & Tulasiewicz, 1995). However, as Fish (1995) points out, if mentoring is considered in its more enabling and embracing form to support the development of independent practitioners, it becomes more in tune with its more classical role.

Since Project 2000 implementation, 'mentors' have had to be more challenging in approach and to take on the attributes of the 'critical friend' rather than provide a more comfortable, traditionally supportive relationship (Cameron-Jones & O'Hara, 1996). This suggests that true mentoring in its classical sense was not in evidence in such an inquiry, and what currently exist for student nurses are indeed the pseudo-mentoring approaches which do not challenge in quite the same manner (Earnshaw, 1995).

There is growing recognition of the need for more focused research studies, 'complemented by the development of a forum for sharing research concerns, processes and findings' (Maggs, 1994, p. 27). Perhaps then we will have the evidence for the depth of analysis which will illuminate more clearly the differences between these complementary, enabling relationships.

In distinguishing between some structured support systems, which include mentoring, preceptorship and clinical supervision, Bond and Holland (1998, p. 20) note the historical burden of confusion and ask the question, 'How is clinical supervision similar to and how is it different from these and other more informal support schemes?' A useful overview is provided in relation to the main structured support roles evident in clinical practice, and mentoring, preceptorship, supervised practice, peer support and clinical supervision are carefully considered through the identification of distinguishing criteria that include the practitioner, time period, how widespread they are and assessment function (Bond & Holland, 1998, p. 20, Table 1.1).

In recognising distinctions of seniority and experience within the clinical supervision alliance, Bond and Holland consider clinical supervision as an interactive partnership with less of a 'power divide' between those within the relationship, than say those of the mentor–mentee relationship. We would agree to some extent that there may initially be a difference in power at the start of a mentoring relationship, particularly with classical mentoring. However, the essence of the partnership results in an eventual balance of equality and reciprocity (Standing, 1999). It should also be recognised that Bond and Holland were contemplating the situation where mentoring is mainly provided for students in pre-registration programmes and where the resulting power divide within this type of pseudo-mentoring relationship may be more evident and remain through the life span of the relationship.

As Holloway and Whyte (1994) comment, mentoring is not the tutor–student relationship where the focus is the course content; neither is it the instructor–trainee relationship where the primary emphasis is on learning and the application of new skills. In these examples it is the tutor or course instructor who remains in control of the learning process. Mentoring should not be confused with the manager–employee relationship where role relationships and task orientation may make it difficult to ensure effective mentoring in practice. Mentoring is also more than a friend to friend or peer relationship, where the focus may remain at the personal development level without due consideration for organisational or institutional matters.

Mentoring is different from other collegial relationships; there are those who consider that the mentor has greater social and intellectual status initially than the mentee, while a colleague is of equal status and the relationship that forms between colleagues is one of equality from the start (Reohr, 1981). In its classical sense mentoring provides a helicopter view, offering the broader picture of organisational and professional life and facilitating development and experience that cannot be obtained elsewhere. It is in this sense a more distant relationship; although it may indeed be more emotionally intense, there may not be the need for regular meetings, and the interactions that do occur are shaped by the individuals concerned.

Mentoring is considered to offer a long term dimension to the needs of both the individual and the organisation; as Conway (1996) reports, 'studies of best practice show that it is more open-ended and less directed towards immediate work tasks and goals than other relationships such as coaching'. Mentoring, it is also noted, relates to the 'longer-term acquisition and application of skills in a developing career' (Parsloe, 1995, p. 73).

This is somewhat different to the way clinical supervision is currently emerging in the literature generally, and in Trusts' policies in particular, where there is clear identification of the need for regular meetings and a well defined and clinically focused partnership. Clinical supervision draws attention to the issues of clinical practice – the quality imperatives, organisational demands, personal self-management and ethical issues that may arise in everyday practice.

The relevant aspects or relative tasks of clinical supervision (normative, formative and restorative) are linked and in some contexts clearly related to, and focused on, the specific needs of the individual and the organisation. The restorative task facilitates the discharging of emotions and recharging of energies, the formative tasks that of developing skills and enhancing understanding, and the normative tasks ensure the identification and self-assessment of professional and ethical competence. This balance of enabling and ensuring functions captures the 'dual nature' of clinical supervision (Brown & Bourne, 1996) and it is important here to reinforce that the normative task is essential to effective clinical supervision and need not necessarily relate to 'competencies', but reinforces the need for creativity embodied within 'good practice'.

Building on the work of the previous edition, a continuum is proposed in figure 5.4 which outlines the various interpretations of the three main roles being discussed here, in relation to staff grade, degree of socialisation and emotional support identified. As Bond and Holland (1998, p. 22) reinforce, it is helpful to consider structured supports as 'more of a continuum rather than acting as appendages or a substitute for each other'. It is of course not as straightforward as the line diagram and continuum approach would suggest, as the relationships interact and overlap as the various role boundaries are altered and shaped by the nature of the clinical application and the cultural perspectives of the differing health tribes. What is important is the balance of enabling and ensuring tasks and that all staff should have access to some form of support which may well include clinical supervision for qualified staff (registered practitioners) and coaching supervision for unqualified staff (students and health care assistants).

As discussed in Chapter 4, coaching supervision is suggested as a useful interpretation of clinical supervision, to demonstrate the inclusion of

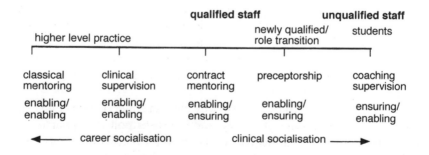

Fig. 5.4 Proposed continuum of the interrelationship of significant roles.

training supervision approaches more likely to be associated with ensuring and enabling relationships that offer more direction than that envisaged within mentoring or clinical supervision relationships.

Classical mentoring and clinical supervision as they are currently emerging in the British nursing literature appear towards the enabling end of the continuum, whilst contract mentoring and preceptorship have enabling tasks, but the practitioners' status and organisational requirements may introduce and shape the ensuring components within specified aims and learning outcomes. These relationships do still, however, remain collegial and collaborative in approach and provide for effective, interactive partnerships.

The continuum as presented also identifies the span of significant support roles and relationships that encourage learning in practice, which should continue throughout all stages of a practitioner's career. It is indeed right and proper that the:

> 'introduction to a process of clinical supervision should begin in professional training and education and as an integral part of professional development.'

> (Butterworth, 1998, p. 13)

It is essential to note that a practitioner may commence professional practice with the assistance of a preceptor who orientates and facilitates transition to a new role or situation. This relationship may then naturally develop or those involved may be expected to engage in a clinical supervisory relationship that maintains the focus on self-development and practice issues. If, over time, the relationship becomes reciprocally intense and multifaceted with the application of a range of helper functions such as networking, sponsorship and teaching, and those other essential aspects associated with mentoring are offered, then the resulting relationship subtly shifts towards that of classical mentoring.

A summary of the differences between mentoring, preceptorship and clinical supervision are given in Table 5.2, where the differences between the three professional support roles are identified in terms of criteria which relate to the nature, function and duration of the relationships that arise.

In beginning to tease out the differences between these complex, professional, support roles, it is easy to see why, in the past, such difficulties were experienced. It is important now that we acknowledge the earlier mistakes and work positively to ensure that each of these enabling roles is given the recognition that it deserves. It is also essential to recognise and establish effective partnership arrangements between

Table 5.2   Overview of the differences between mentoring, preceptorship and clinical supervision.

Mentor	Clinical supervisor	Preceptor
Initimate, personal enabling relationship	Clinical enabling relationship	Functional enabling relationship
Career socialisation, providing social and political networks	Clinical socialisation, focus on practice	Clinical socialisation in initial post-registration/ transition period
Unstructured learning support	Semi-structured learning support	Structured learning support
Long term duration, determined by the needs of those involved	Medium-term duration, determined by clinical partnership and working alliance	Short duration related to clinical allocation, specific period of support
Multi-faceted assisting roles but no formal assessment	Clinically and professionally related tasks, and self-assessment	Specific roles with emphasis on role modelling and rehearsal of key skills
Chosen by individual	Chosen by individual or assigned	Chosen by employer/staff development/continuing education staff

service and education, to ensure that in future mentoring, preceptorship and clinical supervision are located within professional support initiatives that are successfully understood and implemented to the benefit of all concerned.

Recognising the need for a professional support framework

Support systems of a sort have always existed in health care, whether they have come about naturally or informally as friendships or shared confidences between peers, as part of organised educational activities, or the more formal quasi-counselling which happens between managers and their staff. So why should we, the authors, consider setting up more formal structures which may well lead to more expense, increased administration and the possibility of valuable time being deflected away from patient care.

Support is about being sensitive to the human dynamics that surround us and it is also about allowing individuals to be self directive, and assisting them to manage the change process for themselves. By providing a workable 'helping' relationship we can start to communicate properly, build effective partnerships and get beyond some of the limiting attitudes and behaviours which make up a negative hierarchy at work and act as barriers to learning from experience.

Such helping relationships can also assist in addressing the concerns about burnout and diminished staff morale, common to those in helping professions, which result in a range of avoiding behaviours and high absenteeism (Daley, 1987). A more recent study has demonstrated that lack of constructive support in primary care can result in higher levels of stress among health visitors in comparison with their community colleagues (Snelgrove, 1998).

The changing work culture

The current focus is that of a learning culture to assist individuals, organisations and society collectively to come to terms with and to benefit from the rapid technological changes now taking place. We need to be able to make use of the finite resources that are available and to come to an understanding about what it means to live and work in the information age – a period when the following predictions are already becoming an all too familiar reality

- '25% will be skilled workers with permanent jobs in large firms protected by collective wage agreements
- 25% will be peripheral workers with insecure, unskilled and badly paid jobs, whose work schedules vary according to the wishes of their employers and the fluctuations in the market
- 50% will be semi-employed, unemployed, or marginalised workers, doing occasional or seasonal work or odd jobs'.

(Gorz, 1989)

In such an age rapid change is inevitable and competition for resources high, and personal work patterns and consumer expectations will be vastly different from those of previous generations, resulting in greater emphasis on flattened management structures, downsizing and part-time working (Foster, 1996)

In response to the changes different countries have identified their priorities and strategies for better informed societies, by devising projects or legislation that have led to initiatives for greater participation in higher education. In the UK there is a recognised need to keep pace with what is happening and to implement policies for economic growth that will affect productivity and increase consumer confidence (Ball, 1992).

As explored in Chapter 1, the complexities of the modern world require those involved in service organisations to respond to the challenges of working and learning more flexibly. Increasing globalisation, technological advances and economic competitiveness have led to demands for continuing education, transferable skills, flexible career patterns and work-based learning (DfEE, 1995). The response to such demands has led to deliberations on the need to create a learning society and learning organisations which shift the emphasis towards individuals taking personal responsibility and ownership for their continued professional education through processes of mutual, open dialogue and learning together (Casto & Julia, 1994; Leathard, 1994; Ovretveit *et al.*, 1997; SCOPME, 1999).

A significant proportion of the health care professions and other occupational groups are working on strategies to encourage continuing professional development, and more recently those in the complementary therapies have also begun to recognise the need for more formal mechanisms to develop and support practitioners in the field (MacPherson, 1997).

The changing nature of health care – the case for support

Health care is becoming increasingly more complex and expensive to deliver and for staff coming to terms with the market advancements of recent years, a new government and a flurry of policy initiatives have subtly altered the balance towards collaborative practice and the delivery of quality care (DoH, 1997). The emphasis is supposedly towards a return to the consensus management of the early 1980s but the effects of general management have taken a strong foothold and many wait to see what the real effects of the new policies will be. The principles of efficiency, effectiveness and value for money remain in the NHS as those working in the service and those being treated are steadily coming to terms with the changes that are envisaged.

The demands of new technology, innovative treatments and the newly proposed community initiatives are ever increasing (Pietroni, 1996). The patient as a consumer has had steadily rising expectations since the introduction of 'citizen's rights', and the resulting consumerism has added to the burdens on practitioners (DoH, 1992). The implications of rapid change and increasing challenges have begun to test even the most experienced health care practitioners, with many health service staff feeling that they are being carried along on an unstoppable tide of change and confusion (Hughes & Pengelly, 1997; Morton-Cooper & Bamford, 1997).

In an era of rapid change and re-orientation to new thinking and acting, people have a natural tendency to feel uncertain. As Broome

(1990) explains, it is the balance of the individual's internal state and skill, and the support and encouragement that they receive from their surroundings, that will determine their capacity to deal with uncertainty:

> 'If individuals are put under too much pressure they will resist change, but if they are part of an organisation that values change, then they are more likely to take risks and to contribute more to the change effect'.

(Broome, 1990, p. 48)

It is important at a time of such challenge and turbulence to tap into the valuable potential of human resources and make the most of such resources available – resources that have always in our opinion been the health service's greatest assets. It would also appear sensible to draw on the principles of individual potential and motivation explored in the previous chapters, to provide supportive frameworks that are professional in approach as well as enabling and flexible in meeting the needs of both the individual and the organisation.

It is also vital to consider supportive relationships, whereby care workers and professional practitioners can feel free to develop at their own rate and in their own terms. This can be achieved by devising a range of professional support mechanisms that will encourage individual potential and personal development, by offering caring assistance that facilitates the sharing of relevant expertise and appropriate standards of care. Such mechanisms or frameworks of support, involving the range of professional roles and relationships available, will it is suggested enhance motivation, encourage creativity, stimulate risk taking, nurture developing leadership qualities and benefit patient care.

The challenge is to take the initiative and prepare an effective case for strengthening existing support frameworks and developing new ones as part of the ongoing debate concerning the need for continuing professional education, staff development and life-long learning. The route is not an easy one as budgets have to be managed and it is not always easy to demonstrate the effects and benefits of particular support roles and relationships, as those who have attempted this in evaluating clinical supervision will no doubt testify (Butterworth *et al.*, 1996; Bishop, 1998).

The ethos of value for money, cost effectiveness and 'proof of worth' through clinical audit and evidence-based practice has continued to have an impact and current Trust reorganisations must also be having an effect on management systems and staff morale. We are happy to report that we were premature in the first edition in lamenting 'the continuing demise of the NHS', but, as we wrote at that time, 'the patient remains fragile and should not be removed from the seriously ill list too soon'. What is much more positive is that there is a growing sense that new ideas and the identification of good practice can be shared across Trusts and professional boundaries, and this has the potential for welcomed benefits for staff and ultimately those they care for (Palmer & Wilson, 1997).

However, sound arguments will still have to be used to convince the managers, stakeholders and providers that establishing formal, professional support frameworks will bring benefits and rewards for both practitioners and the service users. This will have to be achieved at a time of increased costs and when there is greater competition for the limited finances that are available.

Professional learning support – coping with the changing world of work

As can be seen by the discussions in this book, appropriate professional support can assist development by providing an ongoing, interactive dialogue whereby individuals can contemplate moving from accepting concrete, factual knowledge to demonstrating their abilities to deal with and solve complex problems as part of their continuing professional development.

The supportive, helping relationships assist individuals to plan their development by:

- Working out individual learning requirements
- Formulating career outcomes
- Stimulating evaluation of role and performance within the organisation
- Building self concept in clinical and career socialisation terms
- Promoting self-confidence and autonomy in practice.

Taking responsibility for their own learning involves placing a value on past experiences and being able to relate these experiences to current practice. Supportive relationships assist this process of self-discovery, helping individual practitioners to clarify their personal and career needs in order to discover their own personal style, and this is then demonstrated in their practice. To make this more meaningful, as suggested in Chapter 4, there is a definite need to relate past experiences and try out and test new learning through experience.

For the professional practitioner the processes are those of 'learning through'. This entails thinking about doing, thinking through doing and thinking about what was done and is still to be done, creating the reflexive practitioner who thinks beyond reflection-on-action and begins to respond reflexively (Rolfe, 1998). Appropriate professional support structures can provide individuals with personal 'time out' and space for reflection.

In an increasingly complex world of work where there are few set patterns for practice and few concrete answers, preparing practitioners via the skills of their own reflections appears a sensible and viable option and it challenges our views on what constitutes learning. This is explained well by Barnett (1990) who calls for insight, involvement and reflection, not learning as such:

> 'Students have to show that they understand what has been learned so deeply that they are able to look down on it and assess it critically for themselves.'

> (Barnett, 1990, p. 151)

To assist these processes and encourage critical reflection, clearly identifiable frameworks are required to make the best use of available experienced practitioners in a variety of professional support roles.

Professional support and development framework

Given the current complexities and demands for health care it would appear a sensible option to provide a professional support framework that is designed to meet the changing requirements of professional practice. Such frameworks should be flexible and comprehensive to include the many different development phases and transition periods in a professional practitioner's career. The framework should be designed specifically to draw together the range of support and development roles that are now available, in order to assist those engaged in the increasing rigours of professional practice. The roles contained within such frameworks should extend beyond those formed as friendships, buddies, peers, role models or facilitators.

It is important to note that such a framework should not be created to respond to need alone as this may cause imbalances for some, and may result in increased responses to demand from others (Earwaker, 1992). As we noted when exploring the provision of clinical supervision, both organisational and human constraints have to be considered when making a rational and informed decision on what professional support roles should be readily available. Well-defined initiatives are required and a continuing professional support strategy that will provide a comprehensive network of support-orientated practitioners. These individuals should be prepared to work together to take on the many different roles that are now available and emerging.

A more well-defined interpretation and enhanced understanding of the roles and functions available may aid in breaking down the prejudices, particularly of those sceptical of the use of mentoring as it is currently being 'used and abused' in clinical practice. The language employed to describe mentoring in the recent past, concerning proteges and distortions towards sponsorship functions, has led to associations with elitism and favouritism which may not rest well within the public service sector. Mentoring, preceptorship and clinical supervision, if clearly understood and applied appropriately, provide effective support systems by complementing and adding to the value of the other roles already available.

A broader notion of support than has necessarily been considered in the past is envisaged, with supportive frameworks to form part of the wider remit of staff development, to aid those starting out as well as those actively engaged in professional practice. We suggest that the basis for such a comprehensive framework can be categorised into four main areas of support requirement, reinforcing the need for continual learning and the effective provision of support throughout a practitioner's career. These areas of support relate to the individual's learning and developmental needs in terms of his/her point of entry and specific changes in his/her professional circumstances. The four main areas are:

(1) Entry to the profession – the student
(2) Entry as a professional practitioner – newly qualified
(3) Transition periods of re-entry and role change – the qualified
(4) Influencing the profession – qualified, experienced and higher level practice.

The support framework suggested matches the key roles at each stage of the individual's development or transition. This match is made based on available research, our experiences in practice and education and interpretations of nursing, midwifery and health visiting statutory guidelines (UKCC, 1995; UKCC, 1999).

The ideas for the framework can be represented diagrammatically as shown in Fig. 5.5. This identifies the areas and individuals for support and incorporates the significant roles and relationships, linking them to produce a vital matrix of professional support. This establishes a social network of practitioners – the collective title for the individuals and organisational systems with which there is effective communication (Walsh, 1997; Girvin, 1999).

Support for the student is demonstrated in the recognisable roles of group colleagues or peers, educational support and clinical supervision. In the first edition we proposed a new clinical role, that of the facilitator–coach, which never quite caught on; but we stand by our thinking behind this, in that we considered that the facilitatory aspect would balance the more specifically clinically orientated and functional coaching role. Following an analysis of traditional supervision it seems far more sensible to support the idea that clinical supervision should span the whole of professional development, as recommended by Butterworth (1998). This allows interpretations and balance of the ensuring and enabling tasks of supervision to come into play depending on the professional status and particular learning needs of the individual student.

As suggested in Chapter 4, a sound case could be made for clinical supervision, with a clear training remit for the student in practice. Instead of our previous suggestion of the role of coach–facilitator, formal support could be provided via coaching supervision, with an emphasis on teaching skills, working with the student in practising those skills and offering constructive feedback (Hawkins & Shohet, 1989).

The role of the supervisor–coach introduces the student to the need for clinical supervision which can become more enabling as the student progresses through his/her education and training programme. In developing the clinical supervisor–coaching role, nursing could then drop the confusing pseudo-mentoring approaches that exist for students, and could stop using the terms mentoring and clinical supervision as though they are synonymous (Spouse, 1996). An interpretation of the different styles of clinical supervision and an explanation of training and tutorial supervision appears in Chapter 4.

In the proposed framework, preceptor support is identified for qualified staff who are engaged in some form of transitional arrangement. The qualified, experienced practitioner may alternatively be offered access to formal support by way of a contract or formal mentor, as part of a formal mentoring programme. These programmes could be offered for qualified staff as part of a recognised staff development programme. A contract mentor, by providing an essentially collaborative and collegial relationship of personal equality, could help develop those experienced, qualified staff who wished to take more responsibility to:

- Develop effective leadership qualities
- Broaden their professional network
- Begin to influence the profession.

Clinical supervision, as seen by the previous discussions, is a suitable relationship to encompass the working careers of most practitioners, but it may also be useful to consider some form of mentoring – be it contract or classical – for those who will be expected to achieve what may soon become identified as 'higher level practice'. In order to bring some element of control and recognition to new roles and responsibilities blossoming in practice often in response to local needs and demands, the UK has commissioned a consultancy team to investigate a sensible and sensitive way through the maze (UKCC, 1999). The term 'higher level' will, it would appear, apply to the current roles of advanced practitioner, clinical nurse specialist and nurse practitioner, and will provide a way of recognising and rewarding professional competency at this new level.

Naturally chosen, career relationships such as those of classical mentoring should be allowed to develop spontaneously as these relationships are fluid, flexible and dynamic. Some specified roles, such as preceptorship and clinical supervision, may extend beyond their identified 'shelf life', given the right mix of personal qualities and enough time and the relevant contact to develop mutual trust and respect, with the result that the enabling intimacy of classical mentoring may occur. The classical mentor is included in Fig. 5.5 to show how it can be available to all personnel in the organisation and fit into the general scheme of supportive relationships. It may be that this will become the relationship of choice for those 'enablers' who wish to engage in 'higher level' practice and begin to effect the cultural change towards collaborative working.

A basis for collaborative partnership

The need for professional support which resounds in the British literature is a strong argument for education staff to work together with in-service managers, in-service support staff and health care practitioners to bring together the strengths and skills of all in a spirit of colleagueship. The models of professional education developed could then be sensitive to the pressure affecting the workplace and the theoretical concepts advocated by teaching staff who have the requisite background and expertise in professional education.

The development of nursing support teams and the other developments identified in Chapter 3 concerning preceptorship have been instrumental in helping clinical and managerial staff to reappraise existing practice learning environments, question current limitations and reassess the prevailing philosophies of care offered to patients and clients on a day-to-day basis. It has to be recognised, however, that limited financial and staffing resources place severe time con-

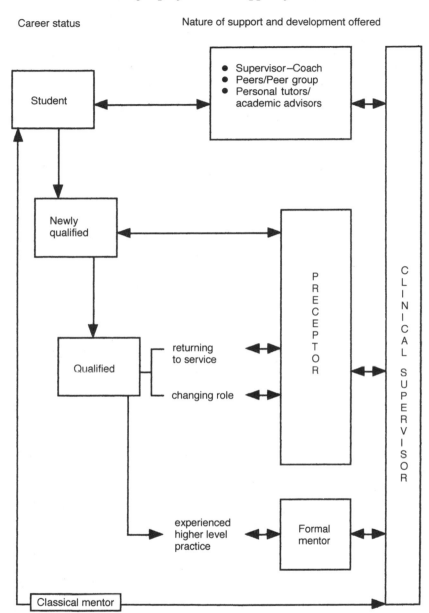

Career status

Nature of support and development offered

Fig. 5.5 General Professional Support Framework incorporating significant relationships and roles.

straints on staff striving to enact change. However enthusiastic or willing staff are to help, someone has to maintain an overview on which resources are the most cost-effective in human as well as financial terms.

Appropriate development and delegation of roles and the need to express fears and worries about the possible implications of change are an essential part of the coping process. Ogier (1989) has pointed out that the raising of staff awareness as to how care *should* be, can arouse distress when they feel that such standards are not being met.

The starting point for the delivery of professional support is a feeling of empathy and trust, and of mutual understanding between employer and employee. Before exposing ourselves to a reappraisal of the *status quo*, it is necessary to establish a feeling of trust and mutual respect in a team or between colleagues working closely together. Because some staff work directly with clients and may only have minimal contact with colleagues, extra effort should be made to provide avenues of support which enable lone practitioners (for example, community staff in rural areas or clinical nurse specialists) to meet on a regular basis with at least one individual who understands and has some experience of the work they undertake.

The apparent priorities for implementing support, as identified in Chapter 3 and worth restating here, are:

- Establishing the policy and procedural steps necessary for the reappraisal of current support systems
- Establishing a basis for partnership with service and education
- Re-affirming the trust and respect offered to and between colleagues
- Providing a forum for support which allows for uncertainties to be expressed
- Accepting the need to explore mutual understanding of professional support roles and to clarify these for any future use.

These are important areas for debate and prepare staff and the service for the changes that will eventually emerge. Figure 5.6 shows an overview of support management initiatives, crystallising the deliberations, ideas and processes that will set the agenda for professional support in action. We would argue, however, that it is also important to consider the quality and ethical implications of providing a professional support framework that is flexible to meet the needs of staff but responsive to service demands.

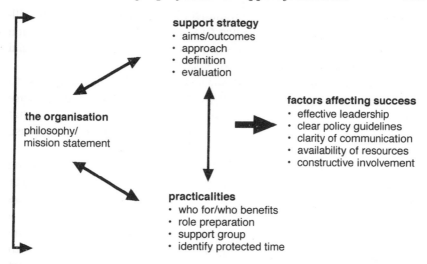

Fig. 5.6   Overview of support management.

Issues of quality in professional support: an overview of ethical concepts

There are certain fundamental questions to be asked when considering the quality of learning and professional support offered to both students and qualified staff:

- Is the support accessible?
- Do staff know who to turn to for help and advice?
- Are the intentions of support offered clear and unambiguous?
- Is any formal support process explained fully in advance and are opportunities offered for questions and clarification?
- How user-friendly is the documentation associated with support systems (for example learning contracts or commitments, mentor agreements, critical incident reports, evaluation methods, ethical guidelines)? Can this be easily referred to and yet confidential of its sources? (By common consent, confidentiality is an important element in health care; patients and clients expect it and so do staff (Brown *et al.*, 1992).)

Katz has examined the developmental career stages of teachers and described the stages as *survival, consolidation, renewal* and *maturity* (cited in Cervero, 1988). Given that those in health care also work within service objectives, direct comparisons can be seen between such stages.

A period of transition is likely at each stage, with elements of all four stages entering into a person's coping strategy at each stage. Therefore it is necessary when providing a support system to be sensitive to the issues and personalities involved. Sensitivity to a person's self-image and work identity is vital, as work identities operate as both causes and consequences of (women's) working lives, and stand in systemic relationship to other aspects of social conditioning (Rosenfeld & Spenner, 1988).

The support framework that fails to identify the self-image of those involved and work towards positive reinforcement may not help adult learners to participate fully in its goals. We need to continue the analysis of the factors that both motivate and demotivate learners so that strategies can be developed to meet the constraints that these produce.

Some staff will consider their work identities and roles extremely important, while others will see them as less significant and therefore less worthy of spending intensive time and effort on. Bevis, (cited in Leddy & Pepper, 1989) identifies the following aspects as effective motivating strategies for learning. Added to the evaluative framework proposed for clinical supervision in Chapter 4, these could provide a sound basis for a critical analysis of any learning support programme. Bevis suggests that the adult learner should be supported to engage in active analysis and raise questions, achieved by supporting and 'nurturing' the:

- Learner
- Ethical code
- Caring role
- Creative drive
- Curiosity and the search for satisfying ideas
- Assertiveness
- Desire to seek dialogue.

(Leddy & Pepper, 1989, p. 331)

These are very helpful considerations which link well with the explorations of previous chapters and make the case for reflection activities to be included within clinical supervision. Just as we seek to develop standards of care for patients and clients, standards or protocols of support should be developed which reflect therapeutic role models in health care. This it is argued will have beneficial outcomes and it is suggested that therapeutic activities could usefully be included in the the implementation of staff support roles in clinical practice (McMahon & Pearson, 1991). Such activities include:

(1) Developing partnership, intimacy and reciprocity in relationships
(2) Controlling the environment
(3) Teaching and facilitating
(4) Providing comfort and emotional refreshment
(5) Adopting complementary health practices
(6) Applying tested physical interventions
(7) Encouraging a learning climate.

Taking the last three activities literally, there is no reason why, in addition to formal support relationships, relaxation therapies and good, plain friendship cannot be a major contributor to the development of a positive and conducive learning environment. The power of laughter and a sense of humour to diffuse tension and regain perspective is well recognised in the management of stress and awkward situations (Nash, 1988).

Looking forward

So what lies ahead? What directions will and should those who are contemplating developing or re-evaluating professional support take? What aspects should we concentrate on and what will the future hold? We do not have a crystal ball but there are indicators for the future. There will be a need for the identified roles and relationships to adapt to the changing contexts and increasing role demands of health care, and it will be interesting to see how mentoring, preceptorship and clinical supervision develop.

We would expect clinical supervision to consolidate its place within the continuum of professional support relationships and perhaps become a shared activity with other professional groups in the health service – through group supervision and other joint initiatives. Whether preceptorship will retain its 'transitional role support' definition or will be adapted for a more functional and developing role for students in practice, remains to be seen. Students, as a particular case for learning support, remain an imperative as they are the force that will carry our professional hopes and aspirations forward, in providing health care for future generations.

Mentoring has survived the 'mentor madness' of being in the spotlight and will no doubt find a place in the information age. As the influence of technology and the increasing use of personal computers in education continue to gather momentum, there will be a need for 'electronic critical friends' to support and challenge across hyperspace – the time of the 'media mentor' will have arrived.

In more general terms the redressing of the balance between competition and collaboration will continue (DoH, 1998). As explored in
earlier chapters, health care practitioners such as social workers,
therapists and those working in mental health are beginning to develop
support frameworks mainly centred around developmental and supervisory roles. However, professional support developments for nurses
and GPs have taken different directions, with support for nurses being
increasingly provided through clinical supervision and for GPs through
continuing professional education. The latter has been revealed as
inadequate, in the context of the London Inner Zone – Education
Initiatives (LIZ–EI), and there is increasingly greater emphasis on mentoring as an effective learning support strategy for doctors (SCOPME,
1998; Wilson, 1998).

That such support developments remain uniprofessionally focused is
paradoxical at a time when policy developments require new forms of
thinking about integrated support roles and processes, in the context of
needs for greater collaboration across the professions. The introduction
of primary care groups in the Government's white paper has raised
tensions among disciplines as more effective collaboration and team
working becomes a necessary reality (Gardener, 1998; Tavabie, 1999).
The development of Health Action Zones (NHS Executive, 1997) creates
an opportunity for members of the health and social sectors to work
together to develop user-centred approaches to care and address the
differences between the various disciplines.

The professional tribes of health can no longer remain within their
rigid boundaries of individual professional accountability to the detriment of patient care (Beattie, 1994; Leathard, 1994; Sprately & Pietroni,
1994). Instead it is suggested that they should work towards promoting
interprofessional approaches that allow them to collaborate as the
boundaries between them collapse (Barr, 1996; Shakespeare, 1997; Weil,
1997). Achieving this will not be an easy task as the barriers to effective
interprofessional practice will need to be addressed and overcome.
These include the different languages of care, preconceived images and
stereotypes, professional organisation, and a lack of understanding of
each other's responsibilities (Pietroni, 1992; Barr & Waterton, 1996;
Whiteman, 1998).

As professional practice becomes more complex it appears imperative
to develop common support frameworks for those who are actively
having to come to terms with working across professional boundaries.
This would allow the sharing of the 'lived experience' to inform, shape
and sustain the active partnerships that will meet the practitioners'
needs, and provide support for interprofessional working and learning.

If we are to embrace more convincingly the notion of 'collaborating in practice' and truly encourage interprofessional working, we have to move away from the trendy buzz words towards identifying how useful concepts can be translated into the current context. We can do this by:

(1) Making the patient/client/user the central focus for the service we deliver
(2) Promoting a common dialogue about what we mean by inter-professional working and collaborative practice
(3) Appreciating and challenging each other's customs, codes, rituals and languages of health care
(4) Starting to dismantle the barriers to interprofessional working
(5) Helping ourselves and our colleagues to make the necessary con-nections between the various practice and education initiatives.

As health tribes we can also acknowledge that we have a lot more in common than we may at first imagine, and by sharing our ideas and resources we can begin to work together and support each other 'in meeting the needs of those we serve'.

References

Adams, A. & Tulasiewicz, W. (1995) *The Crisis in Teacher Education: A Eur-opean Concern?* Falmer Press, London.

Ball, C. (1992) The Learning Society. *The Royal Society of Arts Journal*, May, 380–94.

Barnett, R. (1990) *The Idea of Higher Education*. The Society for Research into Higher Education & Open University Press, Buckingham.

Barr, H. (1996) Ends and means in interprofessional education: towards a typology. *Education for Health*, **9** (3), 342–52.

Barr, H. & Waterton, S. (1996) *Interprofessional Education in Health and Social Care in the United Kingdom*. The UK Centre for the Advancement of Interprofessional Education, London.

Beattie, A. (1994) *Healthy alliances or dangerous liaisons? The challenge of working together in health promotion. Going Inter-Professional: Working Together in Health and Welfare*. Routledge, London.

Bishop, V. (1998) Clinical supervision. What's going on? Results of a ques-tionnaire. *Nursing Times*, **94** (18), 50–53.

Bond, M. & Holland, S. (1998) *Clinical Supervision for Nurses*. Open University Press, Buckingham.

Broome, A.K. (1990) *Managing Change*. Macmillan, Basingstoke.

Brown, A. & Bourne, I. (1996) *The Social Work Supervisor*. Open University Press, Milton Keynes.

Brown, J.M., Kitson, A.L. & McKnight, T.J. (1992) *Challenges in Caring: Explorations in Nursing and Ethics*. Chapman and Hall, London.

Butterworth, T. (1998) Clinical supervision as an emerging idea in nursing. In: *Clinical Supervision and Mentorship in Nursing*, (T. Butterworth, J. Faugier & P. Burnard). Chapman Hall, London.

Butterworth, T., Bishop, V. & Carson, J. (1996) First steps towards evaluating clinical supervision in nursing and health visiting. 1. Theory, policy and practice development. A review. *Journal of Clinical Nursing*, **5**, 127–32.

Cameron-Jones. M. & O'Hara, P. (1996) Three decisions about nurse mentoring. *Journal of Nursing Management*, **4** (4), 225–30.

Castro, R.M. & Julia, M.C. (1994) *Interprofessional Care and Collaborative Practice*. Brooks/Cole, California.

Cervero, R.M. (1988) *Effective Continuing Education for Professionals*. Jossey Bass, London.

Conway, C. (1996) Strategic role of mentoring. *Professional Manager*, September.

Daley, N.R. (1987) Burnout: smouldering problems in protective services. *Social Work*, **24**, 375–9.

Deane, D. & Campbell, J. (1985) *Developing Professional Effectiveness in Nursing*. Reston Publications, Virginia.

DfEE (1995) *Developing Students' Subject Area Knowledge and Skills in the Workplace*. Department for Education & Employment, London.

DoH (1992) *The Citizen's Charter*. HMSO, London.

DoH (1997) *The National Health Service. Modern – Dependable*. HMSO, London.

DoH (1998) *A review of continuing professional development in general practice*. A report by the chief medical officer. HMSO, London.

Earnshaw, G.J. (1995) Mentorship: the student's views. *Nurse Education Today*, **15**, 274–9.

Earwaker, J. (1992) *Helping and Supporting Students. Rethinking the Issues*. The Society for Research into Higher Education and Open University press, Buckingham.

Fish, D. (1995) *Quality Mentoring for Student Teachers. A Principled Approach to Practice*. David Fulton Publishers, London.

Foster, E. (1996) *Comparable but different: work based learning for a learning society*. The work based learning project final report 1994–1996. Leeds University & Department for Education and Employment.

Gardener, L. (1998) Nurse-led Primary Care Act pilot schemes: threat or opportunity? *Nursing Times*. **94** (27), 52–3.

Girvin, J. (1999) Networking for career planning. *Nursing Times – Learning Curve*, **2** (11), 14–15.

Gorz, A. (1989) *Critique of Economic Reason*. Verso, London.

Hawkins, P. & Shohet, R. (1989) *Supervision in the Helping Professions*. Open University Press, Milton Keynes.

Holloway, A. & Whyte, C. (1994) *Mentoring: The definitive handbook*. Development Processes (Publications) Ltd/Swansea College, Swansea.

Hughes L. & Pengelly, P. (1997) *Staff Supervision in a Turbulent Environment*. Jessica Kingsley Publishers, London.

Leathard, A. (ed.) (1994) *Going Inter-professional*. Routledge, London.

Leddy, S. & Pepper, J.M. (1989) *Conceptual Bases of Professional Nursing*. J.B. Lippincott & Co, Philadelphia.

MacPherson, H. (1997) Great talents ripen late. Continuing education in the acupuncture profession. *The European Journal of Oriental Medicine*, **1** (6), 35–9.

McMahon, R. & Pearson, A. (1991) *Nursing as Therapy*. Chapman and Hall, London.

Maggs, C. (1994) Mentorship in nursing and midwifery education. Issues for research. *Nurse Education Today*, **14**, 22–9.

Morton-Cooper, A. (1998) *Preceptorship via action research; a reflective account*. Doctoral thesis, Continuing Education Centre, the University of Warwick.

Morton-Cooper, A. & Bamford, M. (1997) *Excellence in Health Care Management*. Blackwell Science, Oxford.

Nash, W. (1988) *At Ease with Stress – the Approach of Wholeness*. Darton, Longman and Todd, London.

NHS Executive (1997) *Health Action Zones – Invitation to Bid*. EL(97)65. NHS Executive, Leeds.

Ogier, M. (1989) *Working and Learning*. Scutari Press, London.

Ovretveit, J., Mathias, P. & Thompson, T. (eds) (1997) *Interprofessional Working for Health and Social Care*. Macmillan, Basingstoke.

Palmer, A. & Wilson, A. (1997) *New Deal: New Directions – The Evaluation of 'Innovations in Practice Projects'*. South Thames NHS Executive, London.

Parsloe, E. (1995) *Coaching, Mentoring and Assessing. A practical guide to developing competencies* (revised edition). Kogan Page, London.

Pictroni, P. (1992) 'Towards reflective practice – the languages of health and social care'. *Journal of Interprofessional Care*, **3** (1), 7–16.

Pietroni, P. (1996) *A primary care-led NHS: trick or treat*. Professorial lecture. University of Westminster Press, London.

Puetz, B.E. (1992) Evaluation: essential skill for the staff development specialists. In: *Nursing Staff Development: Current Competence, Future Focus*, (ed. K.J. Kelly), pp. 183–201. J.B. Lippincott & Co., Philadelphia.

Reohr, J. (1981) *Mentor and Colleague Relationships in Academia*. Education Resources Information Center Documentation Reproductive Service, Number ED215-040.

Rolfe, G. (1998) Beyond expertise: reflective and reflexive nursing practice. In: *Transforming Nursing Through Reflective Practice*, (eds C. Johns & D. Freshwater). Blackwell Science, Oxford.

Rosenfeld, R.A. & Spenner, K.I. (1988) Woman's work and women's careers – a dynamic analysis of work identity in the early life course. *Social Structure and Human Lives*, (ed. M. White Riley).

Sands, R.G., Parsons, L.A. & Duane, J. (1991) Faculty mentoring faculty in a public university. *Journal of Higher Education*, **62** (2), 175–93.

SCOPME (1998) *Continuing professional development for doctors and dentists*. Recommendations for hospital consultant CPD and draft principles for all doctors and dentists – working paper. SCOPME, London.

SCOPME (1999) *Equity and interchange. Multiprofessional working and learning*. Standing Committee on Postgraduate Medical & Dental Education. SCOPME, London.

Shakespeare, R. (1997) *Multiprofessional Education and Training.* The Kings Fund, London.

Shapiro, E.C, Haseltine, F. & Rowe, M. (1978) Moving up. Role models, mentors and the patron system. *Sloan Management Review,* **19**, 51–8.

Snelgrove, S.R. (1998) Occupational stress and job satisfaction: a comparative study of health visitors, district nurses and community psychiatric nurses. *Journal of Nursing Management,* **6** (2), 97–104.

Sprately, J. & Pietroni, M. (1994) *Creative Collaboration: Interprofessional Learning Priorities in Primary Health and Community Care.* Marylebone Centre Trust, London.

Tavabie, A. (1999) Interprofessional care: how can we make it work? *Education for General Practice,* **10** (1), 9–13.

UKCC (1995) *PREP and You: Maintaining Your Registration, Standards for Education Following Registration,* pp. 183–201. UKCC, London.

UKCC (1999) *A higher level practice.* Report of the consultation on the UKCC's proposal for a revised regulatory framework framework for post-registration clinical practice. UKCC, London.

Walsh, M. (1997) Developing practice through networking. *Nursing Standard,* **11** (40), 33-4.

Weil, S. (1997) Postgraduate education and lifelong learning as collaborative inquiry in action – an emergent model. In: *Beyond the First Degree,* (ed. R. Burgess). Society for Research into Higher Education/Open University, Buckingham.

White, E. (1996) Clinical supervision and Project 2000: the identification of some substantive issues. *Nursing Times Research,* **1** (2), 102–11.

Whiteman, J. (1998) *A review of the perceptions of GP tutors in one health region: towards interprofessional education.* Unpublished MA dissertation. Centre for Community Care & Primary Health, University of Westminster, London.

Wilson, A. (1998) *Review of outcomes of LIZ–EI Projects.* Unpublished evaluation of LIZ-EI projects. University of Westminster, London.

Wilson-Barnett, J., Butterworth, T., White, E., Twinn, S., Davies, S. & Riley, L. (1995) Clinical support and the Project 2000 nursing student: factors influencing this process. *Journal of Advanced Nursing,* **21**, 1152-8.

Postscript

Brigid Proctor
Formerly Course Director of the Counselling Course Centre, South West London College, and Fellow and Accredited Supervisor of the British Association for Counselling.

It is not often that I am invited to have the last word. It is both pleasure and responsibility to round off such a comprehensive survey of learning support systems in the health services – the need for them and the potential roles available. I come to the task wearing a range of hats. For many years, I facilitated courses which offered an opportunity for a wide variety of helping professionals (many from health care settings) to develop their 'interpersonal and counselling skills'. My wish then, as now, was for the widest range of people to have access to the kind of relationships which were enhancing for them, as they lived through times of transition, choice, change, crisis, or distress. Even now, relatively few people are able, need or choose, to have access to a ' counsellor' or 'psychotherapist'. However, we are all, at different times, 'consumers' of education, health and social care systems. We know the instances where our passage has been helped and enriched by chance (or designed) relationships with 'professionals' – sometimes very fleeting. Equally, we are aware of the frustration, distress or lasting trauma which thoughtless, inept or 'plain mean' encounters can cause at such times. I wanted, in whatever way I could, to increase the former and decrease the latter.

Working on those courses, I had three categories of 'consumers' always in mind. Face to face were the course participants. This was a unique opportunity for them, in their busy lives, to have contact with a special kind of learning. As 'staff', we came to realise that the skill of self and peer management could be consciously learned, modelled and, when asked for, taught. We also came to understand, in practice rather than merely theoretically, that the medium was the message. 'To the extent' (as Carl Rogers says) 'that I can be ... the other will learn and develop'. If we could enable the participants to develop a culture and a climate in which they experienced sufficient mutual respect, understanding, and clear and honest dealing, they could trust themselves to be open to learning, change and development.

In turn, offering such a climate to their 'consumers' (be they in role of patient, student, client, or whatever) often became second nature to them. Those recipients of support and help were the second consumer category I had in mind. They, too, were living each moment of their life for the first and last time. Each life event, often so familiar in type to professional bystanders, might be significantly life changing for the individual. Advocacy for 'consumers' (or, indeed, for me or my family when in such a role) was often at the forefront of my mind. A good learning environment is valuable in its own right, but these course participants were in contracts to deliver a service. To the extent that they felt valued and valuable, they could afford to value their clients and colleagues and even become more objective about their often under-valuing systems and organisations.

The third consumer category I had in mind were those organisations, employers, and systems who endorsed the participants' presence on the course. They might represent public or professional bodies, charities or, less often, profit making organisations. In many cases our taxes funded these, in whole or in part. They (and we as taxpayer) had a right to expect that, on finishing the course, the participants would work better than before with their 'consumers' (even if, as was often the case, the managers involved had no way of evaluating the skill and ability which had been developed).

Since then I have practised supervision extensively, and become a reflecter, teacher and writer about supervision (variously prefixed by the words consultative, non-managerial, clinical, or training). Holding the three categories in mind – practitioner, consumer, employer – becomes a sort of touchstone. If the needs of any one eclipse the others for long, the climate or culture of a working alliance lacks something: humanity or intention or rigour. I always seek to hold that touchstone in mind. Not 'either ... or', rather 'each ... and'.

In reviewing the number of support roles mentioned in the book, I am struck how this touchstone is crucial – in mentoring, preceptorship, clinical supervision or indeed in any of the other roles mentioned in passing. All take place within a working context. All offer opportunities for the self management and individual development of the practitioner within a personal (indeed, personalised) relationship. All require the same range of 'facilitative and user skills'. Urging the provision of any of them has usually been motivated by concern for people, to enable them to develop a skilled service to other people, within professional support and constraints. Yet, under the stress of the workplace, and of break-neck change, each opportunity can be, or has been, subverted to serve the interest of one party over the others. Only if they can be felt, and shown, to be in the interest of practitioner, consumer, and therefore management, will they survive and flourish. The responsibility for holding this tension of interests in the face of divisive pressures lies with senior practitioners, educators and those who have experienced good support and know it to be good.

In the counselling and psychotherapy tribe(s), the provision of training supervision has been the link between the 'person as practitioner,' the client, the course and the practice placement. (After reading this book, I recognise that our supervision has been expected to combine preceptorship, mentoring and clinical supervision.) It has been particularly appropriate as a vehicle, since practitioners will mostly be working one-to-one with clients, and the experience of a personal (or group) supervision relationship, focussing on both practitioner and client, is directly appropriate. Within this relationship, practitioners have been expected to learn (sometimes consciously, but often by example) how to reflect on practice and manage and monitor their work. Although sadly under-researched, anecdotal evidence indicates that whenever anyone has experienced supervision which has been helpful and enriching, they *cannot imagine* practising without. I believe that no amount of talking *about* supervision or other learning support can substitute for the influence of one good experience. That is why I agree so wholeheartedly with introducing a climate and system of really good support in training. Those who have had good training experiences will automatically have higher expectations as practitioners.

Continuing supervision has been laid down as an ethical imperative for counsellors and psychotherapists at every level of experience, in direct response to a particular working context. The health professions may have something to learn from our experience about the skills and underlying structures of support relationships – this book, for instance, draws from many sources. However, I do not believe that a similar system would be appropriate in many settings. Each health tribe and each 'family' of practitioners within each tribe will have differing needs. I agree wholeheartedly with the authors that each formal support system has to be tailored to these needs within a unique context, with its particular human and economic resources.

There are three factors which I would like to emphasise which appear (from informal research) to aid the development of trust in supportive and/or monitoring relationships. The first is the importance of the working alliance being clearly defined and mutually understood by all parties to the arrangement. What the role relationship is called is probably unimportant in practice. Roles, responsibilities and rights need to be identified from the beginning, and to be discussed, made real and reviewed. Identifying the tasks, the focus and boundaries of the work together, the codes and expectations of practice, and the collegial manner of working together – these are the factors which allow trust to develop, where trust is due. Discussion and negotiation (where negotiable) of the working contract are the ways for each of the parties to progressively know and be known – for a climate to develop which takes account of difference and similarity of style, of culture, of learning strategies and of expectations. When trust does not develop, both parties need to be clear about where and how they can address (or redress) the issues.

The other elements which are crucial to the development of trust are dependability and perceived fairness. This means that if, say, clinical supervision, is to be a regular resource for practitioners, it has to be equally available for all, and has to be a regular commitment. It then has to be dependably available when promised. Where less formal support is advocated officially (peer support or classical mentoring , for instance) access, time and place have to be available to all. To pretend to offer something worthwhile is more debilitating for the practitioner than to be honest about lack of support.

In conclusion, I have to own that I sometimes think that I, and these passionate and thoughtful authors, live in cloud cuckoo land. Will there ever be a system which is as supportive to its service deliverers as it purports to be to its consumers? Is it an impossible dream that if I am ill in hospital, I can reliably depend on being cared for, in an individual way, by nurses, doctors and ancillary workers who themselves feel valued; who are allowed regular opportunity to reflect on their work and value the opportunity highly; who are competent, confident and self-monitoring enough to be both safe and creative; and who experience their working life as predominantly worth-while, and personally fulfilling? Is it wistful to think that billions of pounds spent on new technology and information systems might free people to give time and attention to human talents and relationships which cannot (yet, at any rate) be replicated artificially? Perhaps we might as well think of flying to the moon. But we did, didn't we?

Index